THE
INVISIBLE
GIRL
A SECRET LIFE

SAMANTHA HOUGHTON

"The chapters were so compelling that I just carried on reading them until the end of the book. It's really interesting, very readable and you have a really good writing style. It's amazing. What an achievement."
GILL – SPECIALIST HEALTH VISITOR

"Just read this and all I can say is WOW! It's gripping. Your descriptions are so amazing I can feel them. I loved your poems as well."
CLAIRE – RETIRED LEARNING DISABILITY NURSE

"It's incredible reading, it takes me back to my horrendous school years. In that respect, kids are in a better position now. Low mood, depression and self harm are much more talked about and I think there is more sympathy, empathy and acceptance that you're not a freak."
RACHEL – BUSINESS OWNER

"Well done Sam and very well written. I went through a lot of that dark time with your mum and know how worried she was about you. So glad that you're finally in a happy place."
BRENDA – FAMILY FRIEND

Acknowledgments:

This book was an idea for a long time and maybe would have remained just that without the encouragement, support and contributions from some special people in my life. My biggest supporter is my son, Joe, and he has always been the shining light in my turning my life around. My love for him is unconditional and I am so proud of the young man he is. To my Mum and Dad for their love and blessings for me writing this book. The love and support of my brother Marcus. My beloved Grandma for the special times we spent together especially on Saturdays. The female Samaritan that I spoke to on several occasions, for her empathy and being there for me and saving my life. The Educational Psychologist that spoke to me on my surprise arrival, for your kindness and getting me help. Staff at the adolescent unit. My friend Vicki for being a great support in my teen years. My kind college counsellor for the support and getting me through my college year. My friend Louise McNulty for standing by me at catering college and visiting me in hospital (sadly passed away last year). To sweet Edna who took me under her wing in the adult hospital. My long term counsellor for the difference she made to me, the first therapist that I felt really understood me. My dear long term friends Angelina, Jem and Gill for your ongoing love and friendship. Lesley the mentor for the encouragement to do what was right for me. To Lorna Sheldon for going above and beyond in the business world with your fabulous speaker training. Helen for your kindness and amazing holistic therapy most weeks. A very special thank you to the following amazing and kind people for your crowd funding contributions that made this book possible – Fiona Hutchinson, Karen Wilbourn, Claire Ramsden, Dawn Chivers, Romincita Davis, Edith Cattell, Swati Mistry, Gill Jakes, Jane Wildbore, Karen Serdeczna,Suzy Berraoui, Rachel Donaldson, Brenda Kay, Simon Miller, Jo Tarrat, Marina Broadley, Danielle Curry, Dawn Wain, Susan Brookes, Jemini Lakhani, Maureen Cox, David Cox and Joe Houghton. A massive thank you to Clare "purplestar" McCabe of Purple Star Design for stepping forward to generously proof, edit, typeset, cover design and publish this book with love. To Eleanor Whibley of Eleanor Whibley Photography for the photo shoot at Western Park. To Debbie of Roundabout Hinckley for proof reading this book. To John Coster for generously arranging my book launch at Choice Unlimited event in Leicester. Heartfelt gratitude to everyone else that has encouraged, supported and nurtured me when times were not always as good as they are now and cheered me on during my business and life journey.

Copyright © 2017 Samantha Houghton www.samanthahoughton.co.uk
Design by Clare McCabe www.purplestardesign.co.uk
All rights reserved.
ISBN 978 1 5272 0899 5
First Edition

CHAPTERS

Samantha Houghton

CHAPTER ONE
THE MOVE

Moving from a city to a village had a big impact on me and on the family as a whole. I found it very traumatic. I had to leave my best friend behind for a start. I'd always preferred having one or two close friends to hanging out in a large crowd. I found the people in the village to be very different to me from what I was used to. I remember thinking that they all seemed to be into playing the cello and horse riding and activities like this. It felt like another world to me at eleven years old.

My dad's business was doing well, which is why we moved and we now lived in a much bigger house. It was a lovely house and we even had a large spare room which in later years became a games room. I loved my little bedroom, my space in the world.

I started to really get into music as I moved into puberty. I loved listening to music especially on my personal stereo as they were back then, getting lost in my own little world. My bedroom walls were smothered with posters of my favourite band and also my first real crush, Mike Nolan. I did have a very active imagination, and as my walls were covered I felt as though I had so many pairs of eyes watching me! I started to feel as if I was being watched and became very self conscious, even though it wasn't real. I felt too embarrassed to get changed in my room and at one point I wouldn't even walk around with bare feet. What a funny child I was.

I was shy and rather self conscious about many things and looking back my deep emotions and thoughts that I had experienced over the years had sometimes been very difficult to deal with. I tended to deal with everything inwardly as introverts generally do. Not that as a child you are so aware of this.

When my brother was born I was very jealous indeed as I had to learn to share my parents now with another little person. I shouted at the health visitors to leave my brother alone. I felt envy a lot over the years to come.

I had some naughty moments which were born out of feeling very angry and I did not know how to cope with my feelings. There was one occasion when I scratched my neighbours garden gate deliberately as I was angry with my parents and I angrily ripped my aunty's net curtains during a visit as I was livid with my mum and her sister.

Before we moved home there was a period of time that was really hard to cope with, I must have been ten years old. An aunty of mine had been ill with severe postnatal depression, I remember going to see her in a psychiatric hospital. It was horrible. I remember seeing lots of old people and patients in dressing gowns. It felt very depressing and I wanted to get out of the place. Her recovery was slow and my mum looked after my cousin quite regularly for a while. I felt like she was taking my mum away from me, as I had to go off to school and see my cousin stay with my mum. It really upset me and I was so angry with my mum and my cousin whom was about four years old. I loved to write and make up stories and I remember making one up called "Horror Hospital" and read it to my cousin to upset her as I felt so jealous and resentful.

I was an early developer physically which made life uncomfortable and the boys at school made it even more so. Teasing me for wearing a bra quite early and when I started my periods at ten and a half, the first girl in my class. I was very sensitive about this. I felt so embarrassed about wearing a bra that for the first six months I wore a cardigan, permanently, no matter how warm the weather was. I couldn't stand the thought that my dad, brother or granddad would see the bra straps through my top and know my secret.

At the village primary school, I made one close friend, Claire and she seemed to take me under her wing. Even though we were from different backgrounds, we got on well. I stayed over at her house a few times and we would spend hours talking about music we liked and growing up. I felt safe staying at Claire's.

The school itself, was tiny compared to what I had been used to in the city. Everyone seemed to know one another and it was harder to disappear into the background. My teacher was nice and she had a kind face. She also recognised my talent for creative writing and praised me, I lapped up every good word as it made me feel special. That was the only good part though. Whilst I was there, I was bullied quite a lot. I was bullied for being a shy and quiet girl, so the more they taunted me, the more withdrawn I became. They also bullied me for being a bit overweight and for being that early developer. It was the boys more than anything. I didn't know how to stand up for myself and withdrew completely. This has happened to me at my old school also although not as much. From the bullying remarks I concluded that I was boring, fat and ugly. This label stuck with me for many, many years ahead.

My mum was concerned about me and went to see my teacher as I was spending most of my time in my bedroom, alone. She said that I seemed okay at school and that it was just my personality, I was an introvert. I don't think I told anyone how unhappy I felt, I didn't know how to and what it was all about really.

I got myself a paper round at the local newsagents, to earn some money for myself. I found it very daunting but pushed myself to do it. It did not last for long. It became harder and harder to leave the house to go and collect the newspapers and then walk all over the village delivering to the different homes. I felt scared to see anybody and if they said anything to me, or if I were to see the boys from school and they were horrible to me. I couldn't bear the thought.

One Saturday when I was due to go and collect the bundle of newspapers, I totally panicked and could not bring myself to leave the house. I cried and told my mum I couldn't do it and that was the end of it. I felt sick with worry.

I became more reclusive, not that normal a behaviour for an eleven year old year I suppose.

I really didn't want to go to school.

The school had brought in the cycling proficiency for all of its pupils and I had to take part. I worried so much about doing it, I felt that cycling brought more attention to me and that was the last thing I wanted. Also I felt clumsy, being a bit overweight and thought that I would be laughed at, another excuse for people to be cruel. The day came for me to take my bike into school and be tested. As I wheeled it to school, I felt the dread creep over me. I just did not feel able to bring myself to do it, and when I arrived at school, I burst into tears, then came home crying with my bike. My mum didn't know what to do with me.

My asthma got a lot worse at this point in my life and when I got an attack I would feel really poorly with it. The doctors said it was triggered emotionally. Even though it was horrible to feel ill with the asthma when it was flared up, I still preferred that to having to go to school. One day, when I was feeling particularly anxious about going to school, I came up with the idea of purposely bringing on an asthma attack so I didn't have to go. I hid in the little study we had downstairs and ran on the spot until I became breathless and wheezing. Unfortunately for me, my mum walked in and caught me out red handed. I was upset and embarrassed as she then started to wonder if I had done this before, I hadn't. That was the last time I tried to feign an asthma attack.

When I did genuinely have my asthma, I always had to go and see the local doctors in our village. They were very stern and not friendly there, I hated having to go. I would feel really embarrassed letting a male doctor examine me and listen to my chest with a stethoscope. I was always taking inhalers and medicines to fight off attacks. Also the doctor always commented on my weight to both me and my mum, they were very critical. I felt a very unlovable child and that I was a bad person. The best thing about being at home when I was ill, was spending time with my mum. When she was looking after me I felt so special. I felt loved then, and I never wanted that feeling to stop.

I was both relieved and apprehensive when it came to the end of my short time at the village primary school. I felt like a true misfit and was so pleased that I only had to go to that school for about six months until we all went onto the high school.

CHAPTER TWO

MOVING AGAIN

The High School, Manor High , was in another town. So every day I had to catch a school bus from my village to school, only a short journey away but I hated it. I lived in worry that I would be picked on and felt trapped on a bus.

I made some new friends, there were five of us usually in our group which meant that often one person would be left out when people got into pairs. It was often me. I dreaded it being me as it was horrible to feel the odd one out and alone.

Sometimes I would cry at home at the weekends as I didn't know how to be the misfit again. Even though I was now well practised it never stopped hurting. I really worried that it would be permanent and I would stay alone forever. There must have been something wrong with me, something to dislike, to not be as popular. To ease this pain I ate sweets and took to buying them secretly as I knew my mum would not approve. It did bring me comfort and was the only thing that did. One day I bought a lot extra to take into school and give to the others, especially the boys to try and get them to accept and like me.

I bought sweets more and more and would sneak across to the local shop. My mum had been watching me from our house apparently and she told me that she did not want a fat daughter and that boys would not like fat girls. I did not feel accepted by anyone, I was so afraid and so sad.

My mum was always concerned with her weight and was on diets on and off. She always looked lovely to me and I remember her always looking co-ordinated, wearing make up and jewellery. She owned lots of different coloured bangles and wore them with different outfits to match . I loved organising the bangles in all the vibrant colours in her round jewellery box with a cushioned lid.

I knew she did not really like living in the village either. She loved our house, with its big kitchen and study and spare bedroom, and landscaped garden. I think she too found it hard to fit in. My Dad worked very hard in his business as a graphic designer. Sometimes my brother and I were involved in photo shoots for his advertising work and earnt ourselves a bit of pocket money. They were fun times.

My dad made our house look lovely, with modern decorating in the rooms. Our dining room was really contemporary, he had very good taste. We had a snooker table in the spare bedroom. We went on holidays abroad for the first time to Spain and stayed in wonderful hotels. At Christmas, my dad was given lots of presents from his work clients. I remember my brother and I got to open the big food hampers in huge wicker baskets. It was exciting discovering what goodies were inside and we had endless boxes of chocolates to enjoy. He would hide Christmas presents for my mum in secret hiding places all over the house to add to the anticipation. Special times were always made very special.

I became much closer friends to a girl called Lucy and she became my best friend. We spent a lot of time together at school and out of school. I always felt that Lucy was more trendy than I was but we got on well. Lucy lived in another village not too far away and we went into town on Saturdays and did the usual girly stuff that teenage girls do, like shopping and hanging out at a fashionable coffee bar, set within a shop called "The Store".

During a summer holiday, I arranged to stay at Lucy's house overnight, well actually in the garden, we were camping out. In the daytime I had gone fruit picking with my mum, grandma and brother and I remember feeling nervous about going to Lucy's later on. We ate lots of juicy berries on the picking rounds. My mum dropped me at her house at teatime. I didn't like eating at other people's homes, I somehow did not feel comfortable and found it hard to swallow the food. I remember one time, flushing some bread cobs down my aunty's toilet which I smuggled upstairs in paper towels. I couldn't eat them. At Lucy's house we set up outside in her garden in her tent. After not long at all, I felt very troubled and wanted to go home. I really missed my mum. I stayed the night but cried a lot and was so relieved to go home. I felt very embarrassed as to what Lucy must have thought, I felt like a silly baby.

All throughout this time I felt very vulnerable, much more than I felt I should have done somehow, it was hard to understand. I felt scared a lot, and was very worried about growing up and the things that would be expected of me. Such as getting a boyfriend, that really scared me even though I thought I wanted one. Leaving school was really frightening to me, as I would have to enter into the world as an adult and I did not feel ready for that. Finding a job seemed so daunting because of how I felt inside. I did not feel capable. Knowing that I had these worries added to my general worry about most things.

My dad's business hit rocky patches and we saw even less of him. He would come home late and he began to drink a lot more. He had been drinking heavily before he came home and carried on drinking at home. Over the time at this home, four years, there were a lot of upsetting times as well as some happier occasions. It frightened me to know that my dad was drinking and I could not stand to be around him when he was drunk. His behaviour changed from being my dad that I loved to a scary man that I did not recognise and whose his behaviour could be very unpredictable. It made me feel on edge. Sometimes I would hear him and my mum arguing and horrible things would be said. My mum would get very upset and cry and I felt very sorry for her. I could not understand why my dad was doing this to our family.

I really feared that my parents would split up. That was unbearable to consider and I would push it from my mind each time. My mum would often go out in the car during one of my dad's drunken episodes and arguments which became very frequent and visit her sister or dad. I sometimes went with her. I would listen and talk to my mum about it a lot. I desperately wanted to help them both and put our family back together. My dad did not want to admit there was a problem.

One time my mum was especially upset and went out but on a bus, I wondered if she would ever come back and it seemed much more serious. I was so relieved when she did. My brother and I were left with my dad at home and I felt scared about what would happen. My dad would always fall asleep eventually on the settee downstairs and I would try to avoid him at all costs.

One evening my mum had gone out to an evening class, she did several different ones over the years, from keep fit to pottery to jewellery making. My dad was downstairs on the settee and had been drinking a lot. I was in my bedroom and my brother was in his room. Suddenly a big black spider ran across my bedroom floor, I screamed and froze in fear. I had a phobia about spiders of any size. My heart was pounding and I was crying, I had no choice but to call my dad. I didn't know which was worse, having the spider on the loose in my room or disturbing my dad. Eventually he heard me and came upstairs in an angry mood. As he was under the influence of drink, he was in a terrible mood and could not even speak properly. He didn't do anything, even though I was really scared and crying. He went back downstairs in a huff. I sobbed and sobbed. I was too scared to move in my room but was now really hurt that my dad just walked away from me and did not seem to care. After what seemed like hours, my mum came home from her class. I called her straight away and she found the spider and removed it. She comforted me as she knew how scared I was of them. She was my hero that night.

I know that there were many more occasions but I pushed them out of my mind.

A few years later I rang Al Anon for my mum but no one ever went to a meeting.

My internal terror about growing up intensified as time went on, I felt so alone.

Eventually my dad lost his business and at the same time his dad passed away. I could tell he was under a huge amount of pressure and it was a very upsetting time. I loved my Grandad and we had many family holidays altogether with my Grandma as well. I felt sorry for my grandma and I used to see her a lot at weekends, going to visit her on a Saturday. I was very close to her. We would go shopping, then she would make us some lunch and we would play games or go out to jumble sales. I felt safe at her house.

We had to leave our lovely home fast at the end and we had no other home to move into at that point. Someone from the village allowed us to rent out part of their cottage and we moved in quickly for about two months before my dad managed to find us a new home to live in. We moved from the village and to a bigger town and a smaller house.

I got through my High School years but then had to change schools again at fourteen to move to the next school which included a sixth form.

My life was about to take a turn for the worse little did I know. For some cruel reason, the new school decided to split me up from my friendship group. I was in a form with nobody that I knew. My friends had managed to stay together. Any confidence that I did have was destroyed and I hated school now. It was a relief when I saw some of them in lessons but I felt it was so unfair for this to have happened.

After a few weeks, a new girl joined the school. We became friends as she was "different" too. By this stage I had started to get interested in the punk scene and was dressing differently and was really into alternative music. I walked around dressed in black head to toe as this school did not have a uniform. My hair was spiked and alternated between pink, blue and black. I would spend ages perfecting my punk hairstyle, crimping, back combing and set with lashings of hairspray. Once a week I had to use soap spirits to remove all of the gunk from my hair and comb out the knots. I spent hours listening to the music and got involved with writing to like minded penpals. I loved writing letters but I felt ashamed as I didn't have a boyfriend, so I made one up to write about. His name was Greg.

Living this lifestyle brought me some confidence, more outwardly I guess and made me feel like I could cope better with myself and my life. My family were disgusted at how I looked as I must have looked quite outrageous to others. I would distress clothes by bleaching them and ripping them and adorning with shiny safety pins. I loved studded wristbands and wore lots of silver crosses and bangles, even a washing machine belt became a bracelet. My make up was dramatic with a white pan face, heavy dark eye make up and red or black lips. Quite a sight.

I also developed a love for horror films, it fitted in perfectly with my look. I also decided to become a vegetarian much to my mum's dismay. She cooked me lots of special dishes but I didn't really like many vegetables and I ate a lot of cheese and a lot more junk type food. My weight was gradually increasing.

My new friendship with Jess was such a blessing. We were like two peas in a pod and spent all of our spare time together and spent hours giggling and chatting. We must have looked quite a vision at school in our alternative dress. Jess had short spiky blond hair. Her family ran a pub in the village where she lived and we spent a lot of time upstairs in the pub as her parents would be working behind the bar. I gradually became more of a goth with her influence and we were both into vampires. We created our own little fantasy family, giving each other vampirish names, Divinia and Santania. Then we nicknamed other things, such as the pencil case as Cuthbert and spent many times laughing about our private jokes. So much so, we sometimes got told off in class for giggling. We were recognised in the school for our giggling and our alternative appearance.

I felt much happier for about a year and it took my mind off of my worries quite a bit as I had Jess now, we were very close.

One day Jess was involved in a car crash on the way to school, I was so upset and saw her get taken away in an ambulance. Thank fully she was okay, nothing serious. But the thought of anything happening to her and losing her scared me.

As time went on, I sometimes felt a bit uncomfortable with her and I suspected she had deeper feelings for me. I only wanted us to be friends. Not too long afterwards, it all turned nasty. Jess fell out with me and rumours were spread around the school that I was a lesbian, which was not true. I liked boys but had never had a boyfriend and it scared me. I started to wonder if I was gay as why would I be so scared but I knew I wasn't attracted to girls. I felt very confused though for a while. The kids at school were horrible to me and called me names such as "Jif" and "lemon" which at the time were derogatory names for a lesbian. Some people moved so that they didn't have to sit next to me in lessons, I felt like a leper.

P.E. was the hardest lesson to go to as it involved getting changed and when people were gossiping about me like this it was all the more embarrassing in a changing room. I thought that girls would think I was watching them, when I wasn't at all. It was awful and I soon began to skive off of these lessons.

Before long I was missing other lessons until I did not want to go at all to school. It became a big dark fear.

At weekends I still sometimes would see my Grandma but aside from this I felt very, very alone in the world.

CHAPTER THREE
FALLING APART

For the first time ever, I began to miss school. By this I mean I was truanting.

When I did spend anytime at school, I would go to the school nurse's room, in tears and not knowing how to be around my peer group. I felt so alone, an outsider and a freak.

The thought of going to school panicked me so much and it actually became somewhat of a phobia after some time of struggling with it. Amazingly though, this seemed to go unnoticed. My parents were not informed and the weeks slipped by.

I was now fifteen years old and I should have been studying for my exams, my O'Levels and CSE's. I knew that deep inside of me that this fear of leaving school had been growing steadily inside of my head and my heart was full of the darkest fear. It terrified me, I asked myself why no-one else seemed to feel this way and why they were able to carry on with normal lives? Why was I so abnormal? I hated feeling this way.

When I used public transport to travel the small amount that I did, I started to get a fear about using buses too. In my mind, I felt like a tramp, that is the word that I always used to feel in association with sitting on a bus. I felt shabby and worthless, like some sort of a misfit. I convinced myself that no-one wanted to sit next to me, and often they didn't. I hated using buses for that very reason.

Unlike other kids whom skived off from school, I didn't hang around with crowds of other people of my age having fun or getting up to mischief. In fact, I was afraid of people of my own age, another fear. I felt that I had nothing in common with them and that no-one liked me. I was different to them.

I spent most of my secret time away from school in public libraries. I alternated between our local library and the main library in our city of Leicester.

That was another problem for me though, being out in large public places. The walk that I had to take through the city centre where my bus dropped me off, to reaching the big old library building felt like the walk of death to me. Again, I would be convinced strangers were staring at me and I wanted to disappear into the scenery. I would scurry along the pavements, often stopping off at the old sweet shop or the indoor market to buy myself a quarter of liquorice tablets. Even though I felt very ashamed buying them, I was already a large size, I wanted them, they comforted me and it was part of making me feel safe. One time I'd go to the shop and another time the market stall, so they hopefully wouldn't recognise how often I was buying the sweets, the shame of it was too much.

In the library I would find the most secluded spot I could as I did not want to be seen by anyone if I could help it. There was always the worry as well of someone from school seeing me, catching me out. Or my parents or someone that knew of my parents. I lived in fear of so many things.

I did feel secure once in the library however, it was like a safe haven for me, away from the world and the people in it. I was also on a mission as I desperately needed to know what was wrong with me. Why was I so different? Why did I feel such a bad person all of the time? Why me?

I would scour the shelves in the Psychology, Self Help and Health section. Rows and rows of books, looking for titles that I felt applied to me. I was convinced that one of those books would provide me with my answers and I was obsessed with trying to discover which one. I would then know what was wrong with me. I imagined the relief that I would feel, because if I knew what was wrong, then I should be able to put it right. I hoped so anyway.

I would study for hour after hour, often spending whole days inside the library. Reading book after book about the mind, behaviour and mental health. Everything I was feeling edged towards what I read in the medical books about Depression and Anxiety.

Never mind how I should have been studying for English, Maths, French and other subjects on the national curriculum, I could have sat exams in Psychiatry and passed with flying colours the amount of knowledge that I had gained over the months of searching for my answers.

I did wonder if I had other problems too as I didn't seem to fit all of the criteria and had other "symptoms" that were mentioned in other disorders. I was attempting to diagnose myself. Still nothing changed for me.

When I wasn't hiding away in libraries or occasionally cafés, where I would also reside for lengthy periods of time, I would be at home, locking myself away in my bedroom.

Again, I would do lots of reading in my room, but it was here, in my little space, that I felt safe to be me. I spent hours and hours crying, really crying hard, and not understanding why except that I felt bad inside. Most days I would wake up feeling drained emotionally before it all began again.

I used to write, English Language had always been my favourite and strongest subject at school, when I was there. A teacher had once told my parents that I excelled when it came to this. I could write for ages, reeling off page after page, pouring out my inner thoughts and feelings into descriptive pieces or poetry. I found this a comfort too, an outlet for releasing bottled up tension that I found hard to express any other way. It was rather therapeutic.

I can remember having a secret dream of wanting to be an author when I was older, when I would somehow have sorted myself out. I could envision myself leading a glamorous lifestyle, travelling around the world and speaking to groups of people. I had some hope, but I think a lot of it was a fantasy that I escaped to in my mind, to stop me from spending every waking moment in my grim reality. I always held onto the glimmer of a thought though, that there HAD to be some life for me better than this one. This life didn't make any sense to me. Why would anyone be born to feel like this?

I felt like I needed to punish myself and most days I would deliberately hurt myself. Usually on my arms or hands. I'd take something sharp, like an opened out paper clip and scratch away at my skin until I bled. Partly scared of feeling physical pain and partly wanting to feel it. I think I was trying to distract myself from the pain I felt deep within about myself and whom I felt I was. To feel physical pain was more bearable than the continual mental anguish.

Most days I would crimp my hair in the mornings. So another

trick I would do is to heat up my hair crimpers , then press a metal object onto the appliance's hot plates and then place this onto my skin and burn myself. I soon started to have several little scars.

Another strange thing that I did was decide to collect some of my tears. I found a little plastic box and sometimes I would catch some of my tears into this container. They dried up and after time they turned mouldy. It's as though I wanted a reminder of my pain, another way of punishing myself.

At times in my bedroom whilst alone, my feelings would become overwhelming, as though I would struggle to cope with them a moment longer. It felt like my head or my heart would burst. I felt a desperation to share this with someone, but someone who would listen to me and understand. It would add to my pain to reveal my feelings to someone who didn't understand, now that would be unbearable as they felt so raw.

When I was feeling this alone, totally alone in the world, even though my family were just several feet away downstairs in our house, I would let myself think about ending my life. As time passed I would think about this more and more, becoming quite fixated on the idea. It was another comfort to be honest, that if the going became too much for me to bear I could choose to end the suffering. Knowing I had that power felt like a strength but it frightened me at the same time. It remained in my thoughts. Stronger than this thought however was the desire to share my feelings. That was another search I pursued, trying to find a person or a place that I could go to. Once I had an idea about something, I found it near impossible to let it go.

Eventually I found the Samaritans. I took to telephoning them on quite a regular basis when I really needed to. It was hard initially to dial the number and speak, but when I did it became easier to share my thoughts and feelings with them. They helped me so much, I will always be so grateful to them. They saved my life several times when my thoughts became intolerable. There was one lady, her name I cannot remember, that I spoke to a few times. She was wonderful and it was such a tremendous relief to be listened to and to be able to offload my feelings.

Eventually my school contacted my parents to ask about my continued absence. It was a surprise to my parents and they were not happy about it. I tried to explain how I was feeling, it was partially a relief to not have to hide my secret anymore. They didn't know what to do and were angry when I still refused to go to school.

My mum took me to see my G.P. The doctor came to the conclusion that I was depressed and wrote me a prescription for some anti-depressants. I was fifteen years old. I remember her saying to us that if I didn't get help that I would run the risk of becoming chronically depressed. I did not know what she meant.

My mum also went to see the head of my year at school with me. It was the first time that I'd stepped foot in the school for months. It was very scary. I was given some work to do at home and my mum explained my situation to my teacher. They appeared to be understanding and were not going to force me to attend school much to my relief.

So now, instead of hiding out in libraries, I spent even more time at home but I did spend a little more time with my family, now that my secret was out in the open.

I sought things that would comfort me, I didn't have many. One of those things was a music tape of Shirley Bassey. It was my mum's, but I listened to it over and over again. It made me feel sad, but I was fast finding sad to be safe. I also still sucked my thumb for comfort. Not just at bedtime but throughout the day, especially if I watched television. It did make me feel like a baby.

The tablets I had started to take, the anti-depressants, were helping a little but the side effects were not pleasant. I felt drowsy throughout the day and experienced a very dry mouth, as though I could not quench my thirst no matter how much I drank.

As more time passed, my mood didn't lift and if anything, I felt more desperate. I'd now received some medical help, but it wasn't helping.

We returned to see the G.P and she decided that I needed some extra help from a specialist. I was referred to the Adult Mental Health Services at our local general hospital. Not long afterwards, an appointment to see a Consultant Psychiatrist arrived. I was relieved as I really thought that this would be the answer to my prayers.

My mum took me to my appointment with Dr. Cooke. It was scary, but once inside the hospital I felt very safe and wanted to stay there. Dressed in a smart suit and with grey hair, but with a rather brusque manner towards me, he didn't seem to understand me at all and spoke to my mum as well as to me. I felt invisible again. I felt his impatient vibes, he asked me a few questions, and he stated that I was "pissed off with the world". He asked me why I wouldn't return to school and I explained to him the best way I could of how I was feeling but it didn't feel safe to really open up in front of him and my mum. I felt judged.

He wrote me out a prescription for a different type of anti – depressant to try. From what he did say to me and my mum, I felt labelled as an angry troublemaker . He ended the conversation with a word we did not know the meaning of. Truculent . He said I was truculent. He also referred me to an Educational Psychologist as I was also labelled as a school refuser.

I left that hospital very upset. My mum was upset too. I felt exasperated and angry as he hadn't understood me and I felt like he didn't care.

When we returned home, my mum looked the word truculent up in a dictionary, it meant "savage, vicious". How hurt I felt that a doctor, someone in authority that I looked up to would describe me as that. The shame of it. I felt even worse.

It turned out that the waiting list to see someone from the Educational Psychology Department was a long one. I didn't feel as though I could wait for much longer, the pain inside of me was so intense. Talking to a Samaritan on the phone didn't feel enough anymore, I wanted someone to be by my side. I found out where the nearest branch was to where I lived and I went along to the place.

Again, they were wonderful to me. They listened and they cared and they seemed to understand what I said to them. Full of warm empathy. It was such a relief to be heard. I stayed there for a few hours until I felt calmer and returned home.

The calmer feeling didn't last for long however, I was soon back to battling with the overwhelming feeling of despair. It would gnaw away at me, feeling heavy in my heart. I needed to feel safe, I wanted to be somewhere that I felt safe.

The wait for my appointment continued, I felt like I was like a time bomb waiting to go off.

One day I decided that I could not stand it any longer, I found out where the Education Psychology Department building was and made my way there. I felt really worried but over riding that was my wretched feeling of desperation. I turned up at the offices and explained to the surprised receptionist how I felt and that I needed to see someone. At this point, I was fantasising about ending my life a lot and someone had to step in to help me. It felt urgent.

She asked me to wait in the waiting area whilst she spoke to someone to come and speak to me. I must have looked a sorry state. I was still wearing a lot of my black goth style clothes but no dramatic make up anymore, just a sad and distraught expression.

I didn't have to wait for long until a psychologist came to talk to me. He took me to a quiet office and listened as I poured my heart out to him. He was much nicer to me than the psychiatrist had been and really seemed to care. He told me that they would try to help me. The feeling of relief again was incredible. I must have made an impact as within a short space of time an appointment came for me to visit a place called Chester Lodge.

CHAPTER FOUR
THE ADMISSION

My parents took me for my visit to Chester Lodge. It was set in the grounds of the Bridge Hospital in the Northfields area of Leicester. The Bridge Hospital was a big old Victorian mental hospital, in years gone by, an institution also known as an asylum, which housed not only mentally ill people but people that did not fit into society for all kinds of reasons.

It was a depressing old building to look at and it had a definite feel about it. I guess the architecture had its own kind of charm as old buildings had, all of the character that more modern buildings often lacked. Chester Lodge itself, was situated on the end of the site, close to the nearby housing estate and shopping area. It was a modern building which housed teenagers that were experiencing mental/emotional health issues. A psychiatric unit for teenagers.

Waiting in the reception I felt a mixture of all kinds of emotions, fear, relief, sad, ashamed. I wondered what was going on further on in the building and who the other people my age were. Even though it was modern, it still had a hospital and clinical feel to it. My visit entailed discussions with some of the staff there, mainly nursing staff and a family social worker. They wanted to know more about me and what problems I had been experiencing.

After my visit, it was decided that they would start me on a day basis as I was reluctant to choose the inpatient option. There was a school on site, well two classrooms plus a gym and two teachers. Schooling was kept up through liaison with each person's school, with some work completed at the unit and some occasional contact with the school.

I began shortly after my initial visit, it was the week before my sixteenth birthday, towards the end of September 1986.

It felt very strange to be going there and I felt very scared wondering what it held in store for me. I felt afraid to meet the people most of all, not so much the staff but the other young people. There were not many of us, less than ten on the unit.

I had a nurse called Meg admit me. Meg was a largish lady with quite a gruff sounding voice. She was a little brusque in her manner at times and I could tell that she would not tolerate any nonsense from anyone. Part of the admission, alongside taking many written notes, was to weigh me and measure my height in the medical room. This was where all of the medicines were kept. Meg commented to me that I had a heavy build as she was completing my notes, I felt hurt by this remark and thought it seemed unnecessary to say it aloud to me even though it were true. My weight and my build was always commented on. Especially by medical people and I resented it. Did they not think I knew I was big? I was fat, overweight, big, large, oversized, whatever you want to call it. It was like it was what people saw me as, a fat person. I was hurting inside, did they not see that? It appeared not otherwise they would not be so thoughtless with their remarks.

After a couple of days or so, the staff decided that I had to become an inpatient to receive treatment fully that I needed. This meant that I would be staying there, day and night, Monday to Friday, just returning home at weekends when the unit closed. After some time, I may be allowed to go home one night during the week.

I had to pack the belongings at home that I would need, it was quite a lot as any overnight stay for some time requires. It was to become my second home, or maybe my first home, as I would be spending more time there from now on than at my family home. I wanted to take some items with me that made me feel safe, things that brought me a sense of familiarity. My bedroom at home was a shrine to my love of all things horror. I had posters galore from horror films, objects of the genre including a rubber chopped off hand sticking out of my wardrobe door. I felt like I wanted to take some of this stuff but worried they would think I was weird or something as I had to share a dormitory with some other females.

During my time at Chester Lodge, along with the other residents, we were all allocated our own psychiatrists.

I liked my Doctor, Dr. White, and I had a talking session with him each week. However I had become incredibly introverted and found it increasingly hard to open up and talk. So it was suggested that I keep a mood diary, like a journal to record my feelings, moods and thoughts in. I took to this very well as I liked to write and it was one of my strengths at school. English teachers had always encouraged me to pursue my love for creative writing and poetry. I did have as part of my secret dream. The ambition of writing a book one day. This daily diary encouraged me to write more and over the next few years I wrote more poetry also. Also they were all about my thoughts of myself and my life and how to cope with it, or not cope as the case may be.

As the sessions progressed, I wrote more and more content in my diary, some days there were reams and other darker days, not so much. Sometimes the effort of lifting a pen and thinking what to write felt too much of a struggle. There was very little motivation or inspiration on those darkest days. What came about through writing about my feelings so regularly was a certain amount of relief of releasing thoughts, but with that came a deep burden of guilt. Some of the writing, well a lot of the pages, were expressing angry thoughts and mostly about my family. I felt that they did not understand me or properly notice how unhappy I was. That hurt deeply. At the same time, I felt afraid to reveal to them how I truly felt. There was a lot of confusing conflict going on in my mind.

When I was at home at the weekends, the unit was closed then, my diary came with me. Because of the growing guilt I felt about the content, I needed to find a hiding place for my diary as I didn't want anyone else to read it. I had been given a metal briefcase which locked and I stored it away in that in my bedroom. But I became paranoid that my mum would find it and open it so I started to carry the key that locked the case around with me everywhere. I wrapped it secretly in a small pink handkerchief I had and never let this out of my reach. It created a lot of anxiety for me as I was obsessive about it. Even though no-one ever commented on it, I was scared that my parents would ask me what I was doing. Even so, I still worried a lot that they would find the case and open it, or having another key and them being able to get their hands on my diary. I feared how angry they would be with me and that they wouldn't love me anymore. I was very ashamed of my feelings as I knew I shouldn't be feelings these things and certainly not the depth of them. The anger was so intense I'd describe it as a rage and the descriptions I wrote at times were very graphic. The guilt was immense. I must have carried this key wrapped in the pink hanky for two years or more.

There was a time at Chester Lodge that created a stir. There were several times but this one occasion a friend I had made, she was admitted just a week before me, and I were feeling angry about something that had happened on the ward. We decided one early evening, to run away together. We had little money or belongings with us (money we had was kept locked away with the staff and we had to request it) to get very far but we had a lot of anger between the pair of us to fuel our journey. We ended up walking for many hours around the streets of Leicester at night. Talking and sharing experiences that we'd had and trying to make sense of our worlds that we were living in. Eventually we were so cold, tired and upset that we called the unit and we got a taxi home. We returned, feeling sheepish and a little ashamed but we were both listened to more after that occasion. I remember that not being listened to, not being heard, has to be one of the hardest feelings to bear and one which we both had experienced far too much already in our young lives in one way or another. I think that this particular evening created a closer bond between us. It was comforting to feel part of a unit again after feeling so betrayed and isolated by my old friend and other school friends.

It was during my time on the ward that I really excelled at Scrabble. I was sometimes playing up to four times a day. My analytical and obsessive mind could be put to good use given the right nurturing circumstances. I became a whiz at beating the staff and my peers a lot of the time. My mind would be running overtime with thoughts of words and scores, a good distraction from the otherwise disturbing thoughts I had a lot of the time.

We had a few different kinds of therapies at the unit. There would be Art Therapy/O.T, in the mobile hut with the resident Occupational Therapist, Teresa, both in a group and individually. Hours of drawing and painting, attempting to express myself artistically. I always found that I had more of a natural outlet through words and writing.

There was also a weekly group of talking therapy, with the nurses and some of my peers. This could be explosive at times if someone was particularly upset that day.

We also had PsychoDrama for a short time. This was role playing and acting scenarios out. I dreaded this most as well as the gym sessions. A trainer called Mitch would come over from the main hospital and give us gym sessions. This triggered bad memories from school and I felt bad about my weight and size even more so.

Each morning the day's activities would start with everyone at the unit attending the Community Meeting. We would all sit around in a big circle in the lounge. Community issues would be raised and discussed. I never liked these meetings as they could be confrontational with all of us sitting so close knit together. It would feel like you had lots of pairs of eyes staring at you at once, very uncomfortable.

School lessons were throughout each day, we had two classrooms and two teachers, Mrs Turner and Mrs Hatter. Liaison with each of our schools were kept with occasional visits into school, I hated this. I found them very threatening in contrast to the safety of the unit.

During holidays and sometimes in an evening, trips out would be arranged for us. The cinema, seaside visits, ice-skating, the theatre, swimming and more. I really hated going swimming most of all. I felt very self conscious of my size and of being well developed. I remember one of the teachers saying I had to go and feeling really upset.

We were encouraged to do chores, especially in the kitchen around mealtimes. The meals mostly came over from the main hospital on a trolley. They became the highlight each day, even though it was typical hospital style food, it still felt a treat. Fridays were always fish and chips and there were hot puddings most days which I indulged in. My favourite pudding was often on a Friday also, Cabinet pudding I think it was called. I was a vegetarian when I went into the unit but gave that up whilst I was there. I ate too much, when I look back, more than I needed. It felt a real comfort but was in fact the opposite as I grew in size. Coffee times involved three sugars in each cup, I seemed to get used to the sweet taste as I didn't drink it as sweet before. There were usually biscuits too.

I made frequent visits to the nearby shop to buy sweets. The walk down the hill became a tradition, walking past the grounds of the depressing, dark Victorian hospital. Sometimes I would see some of the patients from there doing the same as me, well maybe not buying sweets but cigarettes.

There were always different staff on at night. They came over from the main hospital so wore nurses uniforms whereas the day staff always wore their own clothes. I didn't have a lot to do with the night staff and found most of them not easy to warm to. They used to make us supper mid evening time which was usually hot drinks and toast.

One evening, once the night staff had started their shift and the day staff had gone home, there was trouble brewing on the unit amongst my peers. Some of the young people decided to barricade themselves in the snooker room which was adjacent to the lounge. They used the chairs and sofas and it went on for several hours into the night. The following morning, this was the topic of discussion in the community meeting with some rather displeased staff. I remember feeling guilty and angry, even though I was not directly involved.

Each morning and afternoon there would be a staff handover. The staff that were on duty congregated in the nurses room, discussing what had happened during the shift. A written record was kept on each one of us and occasionally we dared one another to wait until the office was empty, then to run I and snatch some of the notes. I think we were all rather curious as to what was being written about us.

Each morning and evening there was the dishing out of meds, at some point of my stay, I was taking both anti-depressants and a strong tranquillizer. They both had undesirable side effects. We also got weighed each week, the worst part of the week for me and it would be recorded. I always felt ashamed.

CHAPTER FIVE
THE STAY

There were some lovely staff on the unit. Nick, one of the nurses always sat in on my family meetings with Josie, the social worker. Nick would sometimes bring his two dogs in to meet us all. Even though I was more of a cat lover, my two beautiful cats, Misty and Tabitha at home, it was a friendly distraction.

Then there was Andrew, he was a very jolly character and was always trying to make us all laugh with his antics. Never a dull moment with him around.

Esther, my nurse, and Anna were sweet, gentle and caring.

In charge was Dr Henton, the head consultant psychiatrist, but we hardly ever saw or spoke to her.

Eventually my doctor left, I saw another doctor for a while until a new consultant arrived, Dr Dempster. I continued writing my mood diary which was shared with him each session.

I felt afraid of some of the other young people, I was always on edge. I kept myself to myself quite a lot and was not one of "the leaders". I was really pleased when after I had been there for quite some time, that a new person was admitted, a lad called Alex. I got on well with him from the start, he was the same age and easy to talk to. He was the person I played the most games of scrabble with, game after game, he was smart at playing too. We drank loads of coffee too at break times. I started to feel really close to him, a connection, which developed into a major crush.

A few of us used to stay up late and watch television or play music. I must have listened to Kate Bush albums and A-Ha so many times, I knew every word. One programme I liked to watch was "Prisoner cell Block H", I think somehow I could relate to being locked up away from the real world. Before I had come to Chester Lodge, I had even had thoughts about committing a crime so I could be put away and locked up so I could escape the horrible world I could not cope with.

I had to do some work experience as part of my schooling there, when those words were mentioned it put the fear of god into me. I reluctantly did a few sessions at a charity in the art department, I hated it. I was made to do some other things as part of my care plan that I really did not like. I had to go on some trips and make some visits on my own to an educational library type place to borrow videos for my work. I always felt that the two teachers were harsh in their approach and I never relaxed around them.

None of my peers really spoke to me very much about their issues and reasons for being there, except Vicki. Sometimes there would be a crisis such as someone taking an overdose or being aggressive with staff. I was very quiet I guess mostly.

Occasionally there would be someone admitted who was considered very ill and they would hear voices and act oddly at times, such as laughing hysterically for no reason.

I had not realised to start with, but Alex was one of them. He talked to me about the Army and wars a lot. As time went on he must have deteriorated as suddenly one weekend they were keeping the unit open for him. Not that long after that I went home on a visit. I missed him like mad when I had to go home and at weekends, I spent a lot of time thinking about him when I was not with him. I felt like I loved him. When I returned to the unit, he had gone. Gone for good and had been transferred to an adult ward. I was devastated and beside myself. I sobbed and sobbed and sobbed. I was furious with the staff and felt such a sense of betrayal. My nurse, Esther, knew how I felt, as my feelings were so strong for him I found them hard to handle. She would have told other staff members. I had no chance to say goodbye and was convinced that they had done it deliberately so I would not create a scene if I had been there at the time. I was upset for a long time and continued to think about him a lot. One day, a few weeks later, he returned for a surprise visit, much better. When I found out he was coming, I felt that I could not face him or the staff knowing how I felt. I stayed in my room for hours on end until I felt sure that he had gone. I desperately wanted to see him but was too scared at the same time. It was a horrible day.

One weekend, whilst I was home, there was an incident. My parents were really angry at me over something, and I was at them. They were both in my bedroom and tensions rose, my dad was shouting angrily close to me and I thought he was going to hit me. My mum was very cross too. I was crying. When they had gone from my room I cried much more, and was so scared and did not know what to do. I wanted to run away. I left the house sobbing, and ran down the road and kept going, not sure of where to go. I remembered there was a girl from school that was also picked on that lived nearby and we had met up a few times. I went to her house. They took me in and I cried my eyes out to Julie and her mum. After I had calmed down a bit, they rang my mum and she came to collect me. I went home still very upset inside. I went to my room and struggled with my feelings, I was livid with my parents. It became overwhelming and I grabbed a wooden ornament I had, shaped as a giant pencil and threw it hard across my room in rage. Oh my god, it smashed my bedroom window. I couldn't believe it and was terrified, that my parents would go mad at me. I did not dare leave my room for the rest of the weekend except to have a meal or use the bathroom, in case they came in and saw my window. We had secondary double glazing, so from the outside of the house you probably could not tell, so as long as they didn't come in I was safe until I left on Monday morning to go back to the unit. I left on that Monday morning as early as possible and travelled on the bus instead of getting a lift. I needed to be away from my parents before they discovered what I'd done. They usually came to visit me at the unit on a Tuesday evening, the following day. Apparently when my mum found out, she was so angry at me that she didn't come to visit me. My dad came and I felt very ashamed and worried. I was really hurt that my mum did not come but I felt guilty for what I had done as well. It had been an accident as I did not mean to smash the glass. Things between us all cooled down and we went back to "normal", whatever that was.

Vicki and I were told of our leaving date, early January 1988, we were leaving on the same day. I was so scared and absolutely dreaded that day coming round.

We had a joint leaving party and it did not feel real. We had a cake made for each of us and lovely cards that everyone had signed. We went around taking photos of everyone. Even though it had been a very tough time, with many ups and downs, mostly downs, I had grown to love being there. I felt safer there than being outside in the world or at home. I was so sad and felt envious of the people that were still allowed to stay there. Vicki and I said we would stay in touch to support one another back outside in the real world. I would miss this place so much.

CHAPTER SIX

SAME OLD STORY

Leaving Chester Lodge was devastating for me.

Inwardly, I had not really changed. It had been a safe place to be, well it had felt safer than the outside real world anyway.

I was to continue to see Esther, my designated nurse. I liked Esther, she was kind and gentle and I felt that she always listened to me and had some understanding of what I told her. Esther was Scottish and had a soft voice with the gentle accent. I trusted her which was a big deal for me. We would meet weekly, sometimes at Chester Lodge and sometimes in the community, often at a coffee shop in town.

At first I longed to go back to the safe confines of Chester Lodge. It was a difficult transition to be living back at home again feeling so lost.

My obsession with Alex continued. I would send him letter after letter through the post, telling him my feelings.

I felt so alone and so afraid, I wanted a special person to be with and feel safe with.

At home, I would stay up really late at night watching films, my interest in horror films had not waned. Strangely, they made me feel safe. I would be able to disappear into a fantasy world, imagining myself in one of these films really helped me to cope with my feelings. It may sound weird, but they were comforting.

My obsessions and rituals seemed to get worse and checking doors and windows were locked became a big problem and that the oven was switched off.

As I was staying up so late, sometimes until three or four in the morning, I would be the last one in our house going to bed at night. The nightly ritual of checking became a real misery. I could not seem to convince myself that the back door was locked or the patio door. The oven being switched off, even though it hadn't been used for hours was another painful obstacle to overcome to convince myself each night before I could relax.

One night it took me ninety minutes to leave the downstairs to go up to my bedroom to bed. I remember standing at the front door, crying, as I felt so worried and exhausted from the constant checking and the stress it created for me.

From my scrabble playing days, up to sometimes four times a day at Chester Lodge, I obsessed over and over in my mind about words and their scrabble value. I could not seem to stop it, working them out, it would drive me mad.

Leaving the house was never easy, but some days were harder than others. There would be two main problems, leaving the house itself and being able to convince myself that I had locked the front door and being out in public on my own. Both were equally traumatic for me. I would often have to return back to my front door when halfway down the street, as I could not settle my mind to believe I had locked the front door properly. It was painstakingly frustrating yet I just could not refrain from doing it. The pressure to perform the ritual would rise within me and I would feel very cross with myself, especially as I had never once left the door unlocked.

When I sat on a bus, I had some upsetting thoughts about that. I convinced myself that no-one wanted to sit next to me as I was horrible. Even though I didn't, as I was also a little bit obsessive about washing, I would believe that people, strangers, would think that I stunk and that I was ugly and miserable. Why would anyone choose to sit next to me? One word always found its way into my mind when it came to this scenario and that was "tramp". I viewed myself as a tramp like state of a being that should be avoided at all costs.

At the same time I felt upset about people not sitting near me as it continued my belief and then I had a reason to torture myself further. Sometimes a person would sit next to me and that made me feel better and that I wasn't so bad after all.

I had to choose to continue at my school in the sixth form to take two A Levels in English Literature and Psychology. Because of how I felt about myself and of life generally I was not very focussed on my studies.

I found Psychology as a subject interesting but not what we were being taught and I really switched off to English Literature. Studying classics was not my idea of enjoyment as I loved to create my own stories, but there was no option to study English Language.

After a few months of attending the sixth form, which I found really challenging to do after the safety of Chester Lodge. I started to miss some of the lessons. It reminded me of school days, pre exams. At least I didn't have to be there as much in attendance , but I was having to not only try and make myself feign interest in the subjects but also found it very hard to even leave my house. Life was so hard and so scary.

I got behind with the work and decided to quit the studies.

I spent a lot of time at home and I loved to drink coffee and dunk rich tea biscuits. I had developed a very sweet tooth whilst at Chester Lodge especially, and was having three spoonfuls of sugar in my coffees. I started to cut down on my sugar intake and eventually swapped over to sweeteners like my mum had.

I longed to be back at Chester Lodge and to feel safe and secure. My sessions with Esther came to an end which I found difficult and I felt rejected. This made me sadder still.

I had started to go to an outpatients unit as part of CAMHS called Wentworth House. It was here I continued to see my psychiatrist, Dr. Dempster.

When I went there for my appointments I did not want to leave each time. I also felt angry with him for not letting me be at Chester Lodge any longer. I felt jealous when I thought of the people that were there now.

I was still taking medication, anti - depressants, and having talking therapy.

One day in one of my sessions, he told me that Alex had contacted Chester Lodge and had told them about my incessant letters to him. I was being warned to stop or that he would take some legal action against me.

I was devastated and I felt so ashamed and humiliated. Even though I sort of knew I shouldn't be doing it I could not bring myself to stop. Each time that I sent a letter, it gave me hope. Hope that I would be loved and cared about one day. I would wait for a reply but they never came. I was trapped in a fantasy world. To me this was much safer than the real one.

After this particular appointment, I left in a crying mess. I sobbed. I felt so rejected. By Alex, by my doctor, by Esther, by Chester Lodge, by my parents, by everyone. I felt so unloved and alone. I was seventeen and I longed for my life to be over. I made my way to the bus stop, sobbing and my heart felt broken. I felt embarrassed of crying so publicly but I could not hold back the tears. As I waited at my other bus stop in the city centre to go home, two men walked past me and one of them called out "Look at the poor fat girl crying" followed by them both sniggering. This hurt me even more and I could not wait to get back to the safety of my bedroom where I could cry and cry as much as I wanted to without being judged.

My letters to Alex stopped.

September was approaching and I had to make a decision on what I was going to do. Enrolment to any college was during this month.

I did not feel equipped to go and get a job, it was one of my deepest fears. I would be judged in the workplace. I found it enough of a struggle to leave the house.

I had to do something, have some direction, so I chose to go to a college. I had no idea or any inclinations of what subjects to study, if I had my way, I would be back at Chester Lodge, away from it all, the harsh and frightening world.

It was suggested to me to re-take some of the main curriculum subjects, such as Maths and English to achieve better grades. GCSE's had now been introduced . It was hard to make decisions like this when I didn't even want my life. I allowed myself to be led by others. I did choose to take Food and Nutrition as this was one area I had a slight interest in. I had cooked at home before and seemed okay at it and food/cooking had always been quite an interest in our home.

The day came to enrol. I went to the college, Charles Keene. As I walked through the corridors, I felt petrified and so alone. I felt so much more alone when I was around others than when I was isolated. I hated the hustle and bustle of the other students around me and I just wanted to disappear. I couldn't wait to get away that day after I had completed the paperwork.

When I started at the college, it was even harder to be there. It wasn't long at all before I was spending my time in tears there. I was filled with terror. I started to miss lessons and found out who the college counsellor was and spent time with her. She was kind to me and it brought me some relief.

I ended up dropping every subject except for Food and Nutrition. There was a girl in that class that was nice to me. That was the reason I could stay in that class however that was really hard to do so I was very grateful for her friendship. I felt like I was a very bad person.

I scraped through with a "C" grade in that subject, feeling very ashamed of myself for not coping again. Another year had passed by and I was no further on. What was I going to do?

At eighteen years of age, I should have had the world at my feet. Friends, boyfriend, going out, college or career and having fun, like normal people did. I was experiencing none of it.

The September of 1989 was approaching, that meant it was decision time again.

After a painful decision, I decided to enrol at college again. A different college and this time on a vocational course. The only thing I could possibly envisage myself doing was catering. I was going to train to be a chef.

CHAPTER SEVEN
CHEF

This was one hobby that I did enjoy, cooking. Both of my parents were into cooking and often hosted dinner parties for friends. We all enjoyed eating as well and we regularly had home restaurant nights on Saturdays. This was when my mum cooked us a three course meal and my dad sometimes helped. They also felt so special as she cooked some wonderful dishes, it brought a touch of luxury to our Saturday evenings, and of course there would always be wine flowing. Then we would watch television. We dined out at lovely restaurants and pubs quite a lot also.

I had done quite a lot of cooking at home myself and I loved to bake. Eating had become a way of coping with my feelings for me, so cooking or baking was always a good excuse to eat more as well.

I enrolled at Southfields College, feeling scared, but it felt better than being at the other college and certainly than at school. I wanted it to be a fresh start for me where nobody knew me.

My parents bought me all of the equipment that I needed, including many text books, three uniforms – waitressing, cheffing and housekeeping, as these were all aspects of the Food and Hospitality course. My pride was my chef's knife set. When they arrived in all of their shining glory and they were sharp, I felt quite important somehow.

I began at college and found I was the oldest person on the course as I had spent two years in and out of sixth form and college, memories I wanted to forget. I soon became the loner again, partly it just seemed to happen but partly from choice. I just felt so different to everyone else and was harbouring a lot of bad thoughts about myself all of the time which made it difficult to be around people.

However most of the people on my course were nice enough to me, there was no horribleness which was a big relief. In fact, one lad was really kind to me and tried to include me in group talks and I sensed he could tell that I was struggling socially.

I made one closer friend, she too was a bit of a loner and we usually paired up when course activities required so.

I loved the course itself, it was very varied and we covered many subjects which were mostly interesting. I especially loved Communication Skills, Nutrition and French culinary language. I excelled in these and put hours of love and work into my homework. I enjoyed the practical side too of the cooking but found the waiting work very scary as it was a lot more sociable. I had to force myself to attend these sessions which were in the main college restaurant which was open to the public. After a while I did miss a few as found them so daunting and I felt really bad about myself.

Life ticked along, as it does, I felt a sense of achievement through my work and the good grades I was getting. I felt a small sense of belonging too which was a lovely feeling, not one I was used to. A lot of the course required teamwork and it was a great feeling as we pulled together at times to get tasks completed.

Life at home was pretty much the same. My dad was still drinking and my mum got upset sometimes. My brother was almost three years younger than I was and we used to argue quite a lot as siblings do. That was normal I suppose.

I spent all of my spare time in my bedroom on my own. I always felt like I was in my own world trying to make it feel safer as I did not want to enter the bigger world that I knew I was heading towards. I spent hours sobbing, writing poems and my thoughts, worrying about what I was going to do and what was wrong with me. I still sometimes deliberately burnt and scratched my arms with sharp objects and my crimper to punish myself. I felt very unworthy. I also felt very angry. I knew it was not normal to feel like this. Why was I not like other girls my age?

My lovely Grandma had become ill and one day she was diagnosed with cancer. I felt very upset. I loved her so much and felt very close to her after all of the time I had spent with her. I could not bear the thought of her not being around. I bought a card for her, with a rainbow on as I felt a significance to the vibrancy of a rainbow to give her hope and courage to fight her battle with this cruel illness. Inside of the card, I wrote her a poem to also let her know that I was thinking of her a lot. As time went on, my grandma deteriorated and my mum spent a lot of time with her. I ashamedly felt secretly very jealous. This made me feel so guilty and bad. I convinced myself I was a terrible person to feel this way. My grandma was dying and I was feeling envious of the attention my mum was giving to her – how awful was that.

As my grandma got closer to her last few weeks, the cancer spread to her brain and she began to behave rather oddly, she also lost a lot of weight. I, on the other hand, was gaining weight more rapidly. I had stopped dressing as a punk but wore a lot of dark clothing still and had let my hair grow longer but flat and its natural dark brown shade. I did not wear make up and looked quite pale. I had no interest in my appearance anymore, a vast difference from my goth days where I was obsessive over my hair in particular. Being heavier was not fun. I sweated a lot when I had to walk far and my legs chaffed badly at the top where they rubbed together until they were red raw. I felt incredibly self conscious about my growing size but had no desire to do anything about it either as food was the only real enjoyment and comfort I had in my life. I wasn't about to take that away from myself, as I might as well be dead.

My grandma passed away. She was far from whom I recognised as my lovely grandma at the end of her life. She had withered away bless her. The funeral was very sad but I strangely found it hard to cry. I wanted to do something for her and I offered to make the buffet for the wake.

I felt sorry for my dad, as he now had lost both of his parents. I still had one grandparent left, my mum's dad whom I saw often. We were a close family, despite what was going on.

As much as the struggle I felt with my relationship with my family, I could not imagine them not being there.

At college, there was talk about the work experience that we had to complete as part of our course requirements. My heart lurched when I heard those words. It filled me with fear and was something I really did not want to think about, however much I enjoyed my catering, doing it for real, as a job was something else. I would be judged for a start.

One of my parent's favourite places to eat out was a little French restaurant, which was local to us in Oadby. One day my mum told me that she had spoken to the owner and there was a Saturday job for me if I wanted it. I was both pleased and scared but decided to give it a try. It was just for a few hours a week, surely I could cope with that I told myself. I had to wear my chef's whites and I worked all day Saturday in the little restaurant's kitchen alongside the owner, whom was also the chef. Each week I came home smelling strongly of a mingle of foods, it never completely left my white uniform after heavy washes. I did a lot of food preparation, especially for the starters and puddings. Sometimes I got to make more exciting dishes, the amaretto ice-cream was out of this world – by far the best ice-cream I had ever tasted. The owner was a large man, and so was the waitress, we must have looked the part between the three of us. All food loving.

As the months went by I found it harder and harder to go to my job which I never found it easy to go in the first place. I was very shy and the others were not and I really felt that they did not like me. I felt very uncomfortable and sometimes heard them laughing and having private jokes. Were they laughing about me? I believed so. I felt really ugly, fat and worthless. I hated myself. I left the job, it was a big relief.

I was now nineteen, heading for twenty years old. I felt like such a failure and like a baby for not being able to cope with my feelings. All of the time I spent alone in my room, part of me wished I had friends to see and do fun stuff with, like I had some years earlier. My life was far from how I wanted it to be. I read a lot of books, horror stories mainly, to escape my world. I continued watching a lot of horror movies too, it somehow gave me strength.

For some years, I had developed my own private and very secret coping methods. They also felt very silly so they made me feel ashamed but helped me all the same. One that I had at the time was that I pretended to be someone else, in my mind, as that someone else would know what to do. They were a strong and powerful person that could handle life and anything that it threw at them. The character changed several times over the years but at this time I pretended I was a prison officer. I watched a lot of crime programmes and prison wardens seemed to be full of authority and power and very strong characters. Whatever I was having to deal with in my personal world, I would ask myself, now what would the prison warden do? This was a brilliant way to help myself and gave me more confidence to do things and speak to people that was otherwise very difficult and painful.

Work experience through college loomed closely, I had no choice but to do it and had to go to my placement at a Building Society's staff restaurant, where I was responsible for food preparation in the kitchen. I used my secret coping strategy to get me through this as I felt very afraid. I hated it. Having to work with people that I did not know, feeling bad about myself, feeling judged, it all felt unbearable. I was so pleased when it was over. Thank goodness.

The work experience was just temporary for two weeks however, so what on earth was I going to do once my course had finished? What then? How would I cope with that? This was something that had bothered me, filled me with fear, for as long as I could remember.

I got excellent grades after my first year catering exams and began year two of the course. The fear of leaving at the end of year two, which was only a few months time, began to build up inside of me. It's as though the huge dread was coming true and I was getting into a real state of panic. Something had to change, something had to happen to help me. I felt desperate and so alone in the world.

I wrote lots of poetry during this time when I was at home alone. Just a small selection.

The Scream Of The Gull

Feeling hollow like a shell,
On a lonely beach,
Surrounded by a sea of misery,
Happiness out of reach.

I have cried an ocean of tears,
Moods as angry as the waves,
As they crash against the rocks,
Where's the smiles she craves?

The screams of the gulls,
Are the screams in my head,
The everlasting guilt, from –
The clouds to seabed.

The weakness I feel inside,
Is as brittle as seaweed,
The water for a mermaid,
Like the trust that I need.

For each one of the pebbles,
I have a fear,
I feel like I'm drowning,
As I'm sitting here.

The World And Her

The sunshine has gone,
And darkness is here,
Lost in the gloom,
Anger and fear.

Never will happiness,
Shine in her eyes,
Only tears will fall,
As she sits and she cries.

Lying so still,
With no reason to move,
Or pacing in circles,
With nothing to prove.

For she is worth nothing,
Nothing at all,
Trapped at rock bottom,
No further to fall.

The Sun Will Never Shine

The dark pain in my heart,
Is enclosing on my mind,
Snatching away the light,
Which now isn't there to find.

Every glimpse of hope has gone,
Like the sun will never shine,
If you see a smiling face,
You know it isn't mine.

Inside, I feel I am in knots,
Twisted coils of despair,
Knowing there is always a tomorrow,
Is becoming too much too bear.

I wish the darkness could fade to light,
I wish the sun could shine,
And if you see a smiling face
I wish it could be mine.

The sun will never shine again,
Imprisoned in the gloom,
My mind can't take any more guilt,
Because there is no room.

The truth is nothing did change. Nothing improved.
I had always had a deep dark thought tucked away in my mind,
that I did think of frequently as I found it a great comfort in
a strange kind of a way. That was that if my life ever became
totally unbearable I did have a choice, I could end my life.
It did become unbearable, the panic and terror I felt deep
inside felt too much anymore to bear. My dark yet comforting
thoughts changed as I began to formulate a plan in my mind. I
started to feel a little better at the thought, a sense of some vague
relief enmeshed with fear, guilt, shame and misery.
As I was such a loner it would be easy as I would not be missed
from the crowd. One day, after sussing out quiet places to be,
for my plan to take place, I went to an isolated room in my
college. As I sat there, all alone I thought about me, my life, my
family, my world, my future. I had got to the point where I could
not carry on, it had become too much now to feel the pain any
longer. When you cannot imagine a future and feel so absolutely
bleak you know how this is. The end. All I wanted was peace,

for it to be over. I did not want to die but I did not want to live as me any longer. From my bag, I took out some tablets. A combination of my anti-depressants and paracetamols. One by one, I began to swallow lots of them, washed down with orange juice. It did not feel real. It was as though it was somebody else doing it. I took about thirty or more tablets in total. I sat there, in that room, and I began to feel very frightened. This soon escalated into panic, as I paced the room, agonising over what was going to happen to me. I wondered if I was going to have a slow painful death or would it be quick. Would I suffer a lot of pain? I did not know the answers and this swept me into more of a panic. I started to experience very strange bodily sensations which really alarmed me and before I knew it I was going through a full blown panic attack.

I rushed out of the room, not sure of what to do, I paced around the college trying to find someone that I knew from my course. I found someone, a girl from my course whom I had spoken to a few times. In my now crying state, I blurted out what I had done. She was very worried but was very kind to me, and she took me under her wing and we went to find our form teacher. I felt so ashamed, I did not want anyone else to find out what I had done.

My form teacher was also very kind to me and she told me she was going to take me to the nearby hospital with the accident and emergency department. I agreed to go with her. I felt really childish and guilty at the same time for wasting her time.

At the hospital, I was seen very quickly. After I had spoken to a doctor and nurses, I was given a vile tasting medicine, an emetic, to take. This made me violently sick immediately. It was distressing as I continued to throw up black liquid over and over and over. It went on for hours until there was nothing left inside me to bring up. My stomach ached and my throat was very sore. The nursing staff called my parents and they came to see me, they were upset and we cried together. I felt relieved again amidst the guilt and shame of it all.

I was allowed to go home after several hours and I felt ill for a few days at home. My psychiatrist had been informed and I was allocated a community psychiatric nurse, her name was Lisa. She explained to me how serious it was to overdose on paracetamols and I had to have a check up on my bloods to ensure of the level in my system. I was not allowed to take paracetamols as a pain killer for a long time afterwards.

My psychiatrist saw me not long afterwards. He said that he wanted to changeover my medication and that I was to stay in hospital for a while. This time it was an adult hospital, on one of the wards in the psychiatric department of the local general hospital. I felt relieved. Someone had listened to me and heard my pain.

Chapter Eight

The Miracle

So, there I was back in the world of psychiatrists, nurses, wards, therapies and medication. The joy of it. This time around I was in the Adult ward of the local hospital. I spent three weeks on ward thirty three and most of it I was isolated in a room feeling utterly miserable. I spent a lot of time thinking about suicide and harming myself, even though I did not attempt anything, I still found the thoughts very comforting, my escape from this was still readily available to me.

Life was different on an adult ward. I was left to my own devices far more and there were no therapies, just the occasional meeting with your doctor and brief chat with a nurse. That was it. My medication was changed, I did not know what to expect, but I hoped and prayed that I would feel better soon. I felt quite angry on the ward as they asked me to be there after my overdose but then there was no one to talk too. My anger built up over the days and I stopped eating much as I was quite afraid to leave my room also. Some of the other inpatients seemed very disturbed and I was scared of their behaviours. There would sometimes be shrieks and loud incidents to the otherwise uneventful atmosphere. The days dragged endlessly, I barely spoke a word to anyone except when I had visitors. Some of my family came to see me and although I felt grateful to see them I also felt very ashamed of myself and of where I was. It was not like having a physical operation and be in recovery, I had tried to take my life. The shame that brought was intense and I felt incredibly guilty and selfish. They however did not know how I felt, how desperate and alone I felt.

During my stay I wrote this poem:

With Love....
See the pink and white flowers,
Next to my bed,
Touched by the card,
The words that were said.

"We are thinking of you",
Is what they say,
How guilty I feel,
To think the same way.

"It's smartie time again"!
I hear a voice shout,
I swallow my pills
And it's time for lights out.

Lying in a hospital bed,
On ward thirty three,
Feeling full of despair,
As ashamed as can be.

This is my seventh night here,
Seems more like a year,
Another gloomy day ahead,
Is what I most fear.

I went out occasionally to go home or my mum took me to some shops to buy a few things to have on the ward. Our relationship had been through a lot yet she still loved me and I her.

A girl I knew from college, Lindsey, came to visit me and she brought well wishes from some of the other students. My form teacher who had taken me to A&E sent me a lovely letter. These actions really touched me. At college I never thought that anyone barely noticed my existence but this proved me wrong I suppose.

Towards the end of my stay in hospital I was barely eating and had lost some weight. I had become very overweight, considered obese and at five feet tall I was around a size 24 in clothing. It was hard to get clothes to fit which just added to my disinterest in my appearance. During one of the sessions with my psychiatrist he asked me if I had ever binged on food then made myself sick. I had never really heard of this and told him that I had not. However, that day, a tiny seed was planted in my mind.

There were also ward round meetings which the patient had to attend if they were considered well enough. These were very daunting, as you had to sit in a room with many different staff, doctors, nurses, therapists, psychologists, social workers and so on, and they would all be discussing you. They were pleased with my transition to my new medication after having been taking an old drug for several years. They concluded that I would continue to see community psychiatric nurse, Lisa on my discharge and to attend an outpatient group on anger management.

I started to feel a lot better towards the end of my stay, I could hardly believe it. It was as though the huge dark veil had been lifted from me, quite remarkable really. I wasn't crying nowhere near as much or as worried. I felt braver and confident enough to venture out of my room on the ward. I kept seeing a boy, around my age in the lounge area and struck up a conversation with him. He was really nice to talk to and it was comforting. Over the final few days I developed a crush on the boy and I couldn't stop thinking about him. This prompted all of my old thoughts about wanting a boyfriend but scared of having one. This really helped me though and a big mental change took place in my mind. I made some huge decisions to change my life. Well they were huge decisions to me. I had never felt this way before and it was so uplifting.

I recognised that I had missed out on a lot of "normal" teenage years and all what they bring, which made me sad and angry. But now, at twenty years old, I was going to change that! I had reached rock bottom and there was only one place to go and that was up. No more of that old Sam for me.

I made three main decisions and promised myself that I would achieve them all.

They were:

1. I was going to lose weight.

2. I wanted a boyfriend.

3. I was going to return to college, complete my exams and get a job.

CHAPTER NINE
FRESH STARTS

I began to make my changes straight away. My mind was set on achieving and to change my life. I wanted to be happy.

I saw Lisa, my nurse, regularly and she suggested I try a diet that she had been on. I had only ever tried a diet once in my life, when I was about fourteen. I went with my old school friend Lucy, and all I remember was being humiliated at the scales when we were weighed. Not a pleasant thought. I embarked on this new diet and I was eating a lot of protein. The weight began to drop off fast which was highly motivating, adding to the loss I had already had in hospital. I was eating a lot of salads. I did feel hungry but I was on a mission and nothing was going to deter me.

After a short while, I returned to college, feeling embarrassed and ashamed knowing that everyone knew what I had done a few weeks before and where I had been, but they were supportive towards me which was a tremendous relief. I managed to catch up on some of the work I had missed out on.

As I lost more weight, it became noticeable and I started to exercise at home with the aid of a fitness video. My mood improved even further. I think Lisa and my doctor were very pleased at my progress. I was taking an interest in my appearance again after years of not doing so. My mum and my friend, Lindsey, helped me with my make up, as the last time I wore cosmetics, it was in my punk days and I resembled a vampire. Time for a more natural look. I occasionally went out with Lindsey socially, but did find this very hard still as I still had some bad feelings about myself. It was a huge improvement though for me.

One day, Lindsey was at my house, and we were alone. After going without cakes, biscuits and sweets for many weeks now, I was craving sweet food. She was also overweight and loved sweet food. My mum had an electric sandwich maker but you could also change the metal plates on it to cook different recipes. I hit upon the idea of making waffles. We concocted the waffle mix between us and made lots of waffles. They tasted wonderful, even more so after the strict diet I had been on. We stuffed as many as we could laden with syrup and sugar. Afterwards we both felt sick and very full. I also felt pangs of guilt – what had I done? Suddenly I had a flashback to the conversation I'd had with my psychiatrist when he had asked me if I had ever vomited deliberately. This now seemed a great idea as I felt too guilty and my stomach was so extended to leave it as it was. I shared my thoughts with Lindsey and she agreed to it. I went up to our bathroom and for the very first time, I stuck my fingers down my throat. It was not pleasant but it brought a big sense of relief. I wasn't sure if I had got rid of all of the waffle so I made myself sick a few times. I felt a bit rough afterwards but very pleased the waffle has been removed from my body, I did not want the hard work of my dieting and exercise to go to waste. I was feeling much happier and loved to see my body changing and getting slimmer.

Feeling my new found confidence, I decided to actively try and meet a boy. I felt lost, having had no dating experience whatsoever, but came across the dating adverts in my local newspaper. Each day at college, I scanned through them in great anticipation. I found a couple that sounded a good match to me and so I wrote them letters. I had a reply, from a man called Michael. We exchanged another letter before speaking on the phone. I was very nervous but excited also.

At college, our second year exams were looming. I did some revision. I did miss some of the practical sessions as I did not feel ready to go back to those. I took on as much work as I felt I could cope with at the time. I was still battling thoughts of not feeling good about myself.

My dieting continued but I was finding it harder to stick as rigidly to it. It was amazing to fit into smaller size clothes and be able to go shopping so I did not want to ruin the good work. I thought about what I had done with the waffles and it became more and more appealing to me until I repeated the experience. Before long, I was doing it most days alongside my diet. Overeating, gorging on foods I desired and then making myself sick. It was very addictive but also very secretive. No one must find out.

I went to the anger management course as an out patient but did not like going and found it difficult in a group setting to open up. I saw my psychiatrist too, he was very pleased at my recovery and also delighted at my visible weight loss and change of appearance. I was discharged from seeing Lisa now life was back on track.

Michael and I arranged our first date. It was a blind date as I only had a description of him to go on and him of me. We met at a pub in town, he was nice. We chatted all evening before going home. Wow, I had gone on my first date, that was a major milestone for me. We arranged to see each other again.

CHAPTER TEN
LIFE IN A TOILET

I passed my catering exams with good results despite everything that had happened to me. My parents were pleased too. It was time to look for a job. Face one of my biggest fears ever. It was very scary.

As I began to job search, I was seeing Michael regularly. He was shy too and inexperienced with girls and relationships. I was glad in a way as I felt vulnerable and a little naïve. He would come over and we usually went out to country pubs, we visited loads as time went on.

I lost more and more weight, shrinking each week but also living my secret.

I applied for an assistant chef post at a local nursing home. To my surprise, I got the job. I had to work an early shift often starting at six in the morning but that left me free to leave in the early afternoon which I liked. Sometimes I had to work a full day shift. My dad gave me a lift to work on the days of my early starts. It would be quite lonely working in the kitchen in the basement on my own at that time of day, but I also liked to be getting on with work without people around me. I found it hard, not the actual work, but being around the people. Some were nice and I made a couple of friends, but socially it made me very on edge.

It was exciting to be earning a wage though, a full time, well near enough, wage. I gave my parents some board money and I was free to spend the rest. I felt rich! I loved going shopping and most of my wages went on clothes, there was great satisfaction in not only being able to buy smaller size clothing but fashionable styles also. I loved make up too and styling my hair, and buying accessories to compliment my outfits. To fit into more normal sizes felt wonderful. It made me feel more normal, not something I had felt before.

My relationship continued with my boyfriend, now officially a couple, I did often feel insecure about it though. If he was late coming over I'd be thinking that he didn't want to see me. I was terrified of being abandoned. When we were out I sometimes thought he was looking at other women. I kept this to myself and new feelings of jealousy were felt.

All in all though, my life had transformed in a short space of time and anyone could see that. I was outwardly very different and some things were on the inside too, but there were still a lot of feelings to be resolved. Truth be told, I did not know where to begin to unravel everything, there was so much. Part of me wanted to just enjoy my new self and life but another part of me knew how troubled I still was deep down.

My secret had become a daily habit, it had become my new

norm. As disgusting as it sounds, it was both exciting, compulsive and very cleansing. It served a lot of purposes and most of all it helped me to relieve stress. I was still losing weight yet being able to eat the foods I loved, it felt a very clever solution.

As time progressed, the secret began to consume me further. Working in the catering industry was making it much more challenging to control as I was thinking about food every waking moment and having to prepare and cook meals daily. Being surrounded by food stopped being a pleasure as I was further embroiled into my obsession. I felt out of control and it scared me. I began to secretly binge at work, terrified I would get caught, then throw up in the toilet.

I had been in my first job for almost a year, and celebrated my twenty first birthday also. I went out for a special meal with my family and Michael.

I felt unsettled in my job, I wanted to change it. Part of me wanted more responsibility as I was bored and part of me found it hard being around the amount of people as it was a large nursing home.

I quickly found another job, more local and more responsibility. It was a lovely private little care home and on my first visit it seemed more like a boutique hotel. The residents were really looked after well and even had a sherry aperitif served before their roast dinner which was served on Wednesday's and Sunday's.

Each day I would be finished by two o'clock leaving me the rest of the day free. The staff were friendly and as I settled in I felt happier in the smaller environment.

At home, my binges were very frequent. If I were alone, I would stand in the kitchen and binge, eating cereals, biscuits, bread, jam – whatever I could get my hands on. I would start off feeling secretly excited, planning in advance sometimes of what I would eat, imagining the taste and texture of it in my mouth. After the first few moments of shovelling food, which was mostly carbohydrates down my throat I began to feel tremendous guilt. Then I would try to switch that off in my mind, knowing it was okay to continue as I would be getting rid of it all soon enough. I found I was able to stuff huge amounts of food away in one sitting, I would get really full but then something inside of me drove me to carry on, almost as though the fullness disappeared. I stopped enjoying the food then and just felt a deep need to push edible items into my mouth and swallow as fast as I could. If I felt that I was running out of food I would panic, so I soon started to have secret shopping trips to buy my extra binge food. I was always terrified of my family finding out and especially of the toilet getting blocked. To overcome this I stole one of my mums cooking bowls and sneaked it into my room. I used to throw up into this bowl, in my room. I'd rest it on plastic bags ripped open to protect the carpet from any splashes of vomit. I was always paranoid that someone would burst into my room whilst I was doing this act. Then I had the task of getting the bowl of vomit to the bathroom without anyone seeing me. This way I felt more in control as I could pour extra water into the toilet to help flush the vomit away. There would be a lot most times as my binges were not ordinary sized portions. It was also much quicker this way as sometimes it took a while to vomit as much as the food up as possible. I'd rest in between a bit as it would make me feel lousy. My eyes would water and my throat hurt and my head would pound. Each time I flushed the evidence away, I would feel hugely relieved. I had done it without being caught and I had got rid of the badness inside of me. I felt cleansed again. That felt really good and took away my guilt about eating. It also took away the stress that had been building up inside of me.

One day we had a family barbecue with relatives visiting us as my parents still often entertained. It was much easier to binge and vomit with everyone sitting outside in the garden where I wouldn't be disturbed.

I got my ritual down to a fine art and was determined to keep this a habit for home only and not in my new job.

The after effects after a while of this behaviour were not so good and it took it toll on my body physically. I would ache all over as though my whole body had been in a fight, it felt as though every muscle ached. My throat was sore and felt rough, my teeth hurt, my skin was not as clear and my stomach would feel sore. It was a very different experience to when you are sick with a stomach bug, much more forceful. Emotionally I would be all over the place and it usually left me feeling low after the initial relief. Even though I knew it was not good for me to be doing this to my body I couldn't stop. The positive effects outweighed the negative.

I wasn't just bingeing and purging, I became consumed with weighing myself. I'd weigh myself about eight times a day, my happiness dependent on the figure on the scales. First thing in the morning, before a binge, after a binge, before bed. I'd also weigh out my food that I did eat and keep down as I had a tight control on my diet still. I was obsessed with counting calories in my food and knew the calorific value of everything that passed my lips. It reminded me of when I used to obsess about numbers with the scrabble score. My weight had plateaued and in all I had lost about five stones. I both loved and despised my secret, but for once I felt in control.

Chapter Eleven
Getting Help

I found that I could not keep to my promise that I had made of not bringing my secret to my new job. As the weeks passed, I stopped feeling in control, it had the control. Most days I would get to work and within minutes I'd be scoffing foodstuffs that I could grab quickly. I'd have a slow yet frantic binge over the breakfast period, in between serving the residents and making a start on the dinner. I'd shut myself inside the little pantry and force handfuls of dry cereal down my throat, spoonfuls of leftover pudding from the day before, cakes from break times, biscuits, anything I could get my hands on. I was terrified I'd be found out by one of the staff but I felt as though I could not control myself. The care staff would be busy getting the residents up and washed and dressed for the day so I was usually on my own. As soon as I'd finished, I'd be in a panic to find a time to sneak off to the toilet to rid myself of the binge. Again, feeling paranoid someone would realise what I was up to.

Many days at work I'd do this again over the lunch period and throw up at the end of my shift. Then I would go home and do it all over again, at least once more that day.

It became hell. Day in, day out, the same compulsion to do this ritual. My body and my mind in a constant state of fear. Fear of getting caught, of gaining weight, of not being able to binge, of not being able to purge, of calories, of knowing what to eat and what to not eat, of weighing myself. I felt so trapped and in some kind of living nightmare. I was shocked at how quickly this had escalated from it being an occasional habit to daily and now this, bingeing and vomiting at least three separate times a day.

I went away with Michael for the first time as our romance blossomed. We both felt awkward at first when it came to intimacy but were in the same boat and sharing a room for the first time was an adventure. Michael did not know about my secret, only that I dieted and had lost a lot of weight. I must have spoke about it a lot as it was on my mind all of the time. We stopped in a bed and breakfast in Blackpool and I had amazing control over what I would and would not eat at mealtimes. It was easier being away, especially being away from my job and being surrounded by food. The waitress even commented on my willpower and tried to get me to eat more, but I refused and felt secretly proud of myself. All holiday I thought about how much thinner I was getting.

Then one day at home, after a secret binge and vomit session, I looked down into the toilet and there was blood. I started to panic, oh my god, what had I done to myself? I had done something terrible to damage myself, was I going to die? I examined my throat and could not see anything. I was so worried

I felt I had to speak to someone, so I rang the Samaritans. It had been quite some time since I rang them. They were a great support as they used to be. A lady I spoke to encouraged me to tell my mum. I felt reluctant to do this as she thought everything had improved for me at last, now this. I still felt very worried about the bleeding though so I decided to tell her.

My mum was supportive and we arranged for me to see my G.P. My doctor was also supportive and referred me back to the general Hospital but this time to the Eating Disorders unit. The forms from the hospital came in the post for me to fill out, some of them were familiar papers, questions about your mood. My secret behaviour continued at work. I couldn't seem to stop it. I did try but it was so compulsive.

Michael and I talked about living together, I was very keen and wanted to leave home. We began to look at houses. This was a good distraction for me and something positive to focus on.

My appointment came through for me to see a specialist at the hospital, I saw a doctor called Dr. Brown. I had to answer a lot more questions on forms and talked a lot in the sessions. I was diagnosed with Bulimia Nervosa. The name itself sounded horrible and I felt a great shame.

I had to keep a food diary. In this diary I had to record everything that I ate, when I vomited, how many times, if I exercised and if I took laxatives or diuretics. I occasionally took laxatives and diuretics and did some exercise but not obsessively so. I knew from all that I had read about that vomiting was more reliable at removing calories than those methods, still not great but better than nothing. I also had to focus on eating regular meals, which I often did but to eat in a balanced way, which included eating foods that I considered binge foods but in moderation. This was very scary. I did it though and the bingeing and purging did reduce. I understood how the cycle was self perpetuating – I would starve (diet), then get cravings, then binge, then purge, then feel guilt and it would start off all over again. It was incredibly addictive and after a time I lost all sense of what true hunger was and what portion sizes should be. It did improve however.

This was an average day in my food diary:

November 22nd 1992

A binge at work consisting of the following – handfuls of dry cereal, slices of cheesecake, biscuit, 1 big slice Bakewell tart, 1 butter-cream cake, 1 coffee. Followed by vomiting four times. This was a mini binge due to no time hardly alone.

Then later on, still at work, I binged on the following – few biscuits, few handfuls dry cereal, few mouthfuls of cake mixture, 2 flapjacks, few spoonfuls jam, approx half a pound of cheese, 1 piece of cake, 4 roast potatoes and gravy, big slice Bakewell tart, 2 glasses of orange, 2 butter-cream cakes, 1 large bowl of fruit crumble and custard and 1 handful of dried fruit. Followed by vomiting twelve times.

I tried to starve as much as I could for the rest of that day but relented and ate 2 apples, 2 satsumas, 1 small bowl of salad and beetroot, 1 tiny piece of pork, few spoons of cottage cheese and 1 diet yogurt. These were all safe foods, except the meat could be a trigger sometimes. I drank lots of coffee and diet fizzy pop to keep me full.

My thoughts that day were elated first thing to have lost 1 pound from the previous day. I thought of all the food at work and was mad with myself as I had to stop the first binge. Then angry as I had to taste the stew that I had made for dinner that day and didn't want to in case that triggered me again. Then I felt a loss of control again later on which made me feel messy and grumpy. I felt very fat, ugly and bloated. I hated myself and was dying to vomit and felt so good afterwards. Feelings of being relieved and empty and of not gaining any weight when I weighed myself. If I ruined a day once with bingeing, unless it was late at night, I usually did it all over again at least once. I was very tired and felt like eating later as hungry. Worried about how moody I must be with people, especially Michael, I don't want to burden him with my feelings. I felt okay later on at night.

The next day was followed by a day of not eating at all, drinking only coffee and diet fizzy pop. On these days, I felt very proud of myself and very in control, almost a saintly feeling. They did not occur very often, as I always felt compelled to binge then purge. Feeling like a fat pig and disgusted with myself. I wasn't even very overweight at this point of my life, but I felt massive.

In that first week of keeping my food diary, I had binged eight times, two days of starving, and had thrown up seventy times.

We found a house and put down a deposit and the sale proceedings started. I was very excited about this, leaving home and moving into my first home with my boyfriend. It made me feel much more grown up. I began to slowly pack my belongings at home. When I came across my old diaries from Chester Lodge I shuddered and decided to rip them all into tiny bits, I never wanted anyone to read them not and certainly not Michael if I took them to our new home. I wanted a brand new start.

Working in the catering job made it very difficult to stop my bulimic behaviours. It was too much of a temptation in front of me every day. I also realised it served a purpose to me and really helped me deal with stress in a bizarre kind of a way. I was not ready to completely stop forever.

Our house sale went through and I left home. I was so excited to have people come and visit us after we had settled in. Each day Michael took me to work as I was now living much further away and had to start early. I began to hate the job and dreaded going in each day, especially after a weekend of being off. I could not control my impulses to binge and it became unbearable.

I caught the bus home each day and couldn't wait for my shift to end. One day, I began crying on the bus. Completely irrational but I sat behind a girl with beautiful long hair. I couldn't even see her face but in my mind I convinced myself that Michael would rather be with her. I had thoughts like this a lot and I used to torture myself with them. As upsetting as they were, I partly thought I deserved the pain. I spent a lot of time comparing myself with other women, feeling inferior in every way. I became very jealous when I was with Michael. It was horrible and I felt so bad inside.

Settling into our new home was exciting as well, being independent and having space as an adult. It was a real novelty to do chores at first, they even seemed interesting, as they were in our own home. It was all new. I felt so proud going food shopping together for the first few times. The whole house needed decorating and bit by bit we tackled it. Life became a blur of work, decorating, my bulimia and battling my inner demons.

I kept having periods of intense pain in my side and feeling really sick. I was scared that I had done some kind of permanent damage to myself. On a few occasions, I had to go to casualty, often at night as the pain was unbearable. At first they could not find anything on my scans, but as the pain persisted they did further tests. I was diagnosed with gallstones and was given a date for an operation.

I was worried that it was my fault, and that I would be found out. The doctors were surprised at how young I was to have this illness and put it down to the large amount of cheese that I ate. I eventually had keyhole surgery and was relieved to have time off of work to recover. They found several small gallstones when they removed my gallbladder. I was actually too scared to throw up afterwards for a while as thought I may cause further damage, eventually though the impulse became too strong and I very gingerly vomited after a smallish binge. I realised how out of control I was with it.

After being back at work for a short while and being back in the cycle of the habit, I got to the point where I felt that I could not stand it any longer. My days were consumed with it and I felt like I was going mad.

I told Michael how I felt and he didn't want me to give it up with having a new mortgage. I understood but also knew that I was at the end of my tether. I could not face it any longer and I quit.

CHAPTER TWELVE

TURBULENT TWENTIES

My last grandparent, my granddad died. It was sad to think that I had lost all of my grandparents now.

I experienced similar feelings of jealousy as to when my grandma died. My mum was grieving for her father but I still felt jealous. I felt so ashamed.

I read as much as I could about Bulimia to try and cope better with my feelings which would sometimes feel over bearing.

I had to find a new job and fast and felt very pressured by Michael. I went along to an agency and they found me a job, I did it for a day. I felt so unhappy and unable to cope.

This was just the start of my erratic saga with jobs. I then found another catering job, I did not know what else to do. It was not what I wanted to do with my illness but we had the financial worries now we had the house to pay for. I felt ever so guilty for not coping again. I lasted in the job just a few weeks before leaving in shame.

Christmas was looming, and I had an interview at an Optician's near to where I now lived. I got the job and was due to start in the new year. I was pleased to have the Christmas to have time to myself away from a work environment to try and get myself together.

I had seen my new G.P and had been referred for Psychodynamic Psychotherapy, I was distraught to discover it was a two year waiting list after my assessment appointment.

Christmas was not easy with all of the extra food around, in abundance. Aside from the fantasy of bingeing and the first few mouthfuls of a binge, I despised the illness and the hold it now had over me. After throwing up I usually ate a banana or tomatoes at least to try and reverse some of the damage. Vomiting would disturb the minerals in my body which long term could create havoc and lasting damage. A loss of potassium was one of the greatest concerns, especially how frequently my habits were, which is why I ate these foods afterwards. Sometimes though, it would have the opposite effect and be enough to trigger me into another binge session straight afterwards. It was horrendous.

I started the new job as an Optical Assistant and settled into the new role. I had training and found it interesting. I also made good friends with my colleague in the same role as me. My boss was nice also. I was working with the public for the first time and it gave me a new lease of self confidence. It was such a relief to not be working with food all day. I was still bulimic but it had calmed down a little and I was mainly doing it in the evenings and at weekends now.

I had to wear a uniform in my job, and I couldn't help but compare myself to my friend, Angelina. She was prettier and thinner than me and was more popular with the customers. I really liked her though and we had a lot of laughs working together also.

I had to work each Saturday, with a day off in the week. On Sundays, Michael and I would usually go out somewhere for the day, sometimes to other towns for a visit, or to country parks for walks. I loved getting away for a while, like an escape. I would often start planning a binge on the way home though, and how I would get Michael out of the way for a while so I could do it. If I didn't do my ritual, I would feel a huge tension. It became more about the release I would get from purging than about the actual binge. Sometimes, I encouraged him to do some gardening or whatever I could think of to give me some time to carry out my secret habit.

I had begun to have stomach and digestive problems which the doctor thought was Irritable Bowel Syndrome. Hardly surprising considering what I put my body through. I had an almost permanently bloated stomach, chronic pain and was constipated. I tried all kinds of medicines but nothing shifted it. I could no longer drink the diet fizzy pop that used to fill me up during my periods of starving, as this aggravated the pain. I couldn't chew gum either or eat cauliflower. I did find that a hot water bottle was soothing so I often was clinging one against my stomach at home. Also a little tipple of br worked a treat for short relief. This was not enough to stop my secret habit though. Eventually I told Michael about it as it became very difficult to conceal now we were living together.

We had holidays and I enjoyed them to a degree but it was harder in some ways for my eating being away from a routine that I felt safe with. I still threw up on holidays.

Sadly my job changed, when my boss announced he was leaving. He was replaced by someone new and I took an instant dislike to the new person. I did not like his arrogant attitude as he came in and changed many things that were working like clockwork. He rubbed a few people up the wrong way, and in succession my friend left, which upset me and then the optician left. Our once happy team had totally changed. I got on okay with my new colleague and the new replacement optician but my job felt very different and I was not happy anymore. I started to look for another job.

Life became one big job search. I applied for what seemed like hundreds of jobs, different types, anything to get me away from that place and my boss. I knew my CV inside out and what to put on application forms. It became a job in itself. It got really hard to go to the job and in the end I left. It caused arguments with Michael and I as we worried financially.

I found work as fast as I could as I was feeling really pressured. My bulimia got worse again as I felt so stressed. My confidence felt very low and I got into a cycle of fear again about jobs. I went for many interviews and came across very well and gave the interviewer the confidence in me and was offered almost every job that I pursued. I became adept at hiding my true self. If I had dared to reveal my true self, no one would have employed me, I was a mess. The trouble was, even though I shone through interviews I went to pieces when it came to the job itself. To the point that sometimes I would not even go to the job, or I would go for a day or two then quit, and the whole cycle would start all over again.

I went for one interview at a hotel to work on the reception. I was convinced this was what I wanted to do. I'd worked on the reception at the opticians and I was good at customer service. After the interview we went out for the day to Drayton Manor theme park, as Michael had a day off. I loved theme parks and rides. I felt pleased with myself with my interview as it had seemed to go well, and I fantasised about being in that job. I imagined it being glamorous working in a hotel and who knows where it could lead. Despite feeling so rotten about myself I also had ambition, the two together were frustrating though as one tended to cancel out the other. I knew I was bright and capable of doing a good job but my mind let me down every time. I got the call telling me that I had got the job. After the initial delight of achievement, I went into panic mode and ended up ringing them back to turn it down, waving goodbye to my hopes at the same time.

This cycle went on, alternated between spending time in toilets throwing up, my relationship suffered. I was incredibly unhappy. After several more attempts at jobs, in charity shops, card shops and other positions that somehow felt safer to me, my confidence was shot to pieces. I was at a real low again.

I went back to see my GP. She was very sympathetic and could see how hard I was trying. She suggested that I was signed off on the sick until I felt better and more able to cope again. I felt like a baby, a failure and full of guilt and shame all at once but it was also a tremendous relief. That pressure was taken away from me at last.

CHAPTER THIRTEEN

FAMILIAR TERRITORY

It was hell. Even though I was away from the pressure of work and of trying to stay in a job, I sunk very low. I'd wake up each day crying, not knowing what to do. I had lost all true sense of how to eat and I cried one time to Michael, as I simply did not know how to be. Every little taste of food could trigger a full blown binge and being at home all of the time made it much easier to do this.

My psychotherapy sessions started, my name had come to the top of the list, what a relief. I had heard very good things about this therapy and had hope that it would make a real difference to me. The sessions lasted about an hour, once a week on a Monday afternoon. I saw a male therapist, which I didn't feel entirely comfortable with, but knew it would make the waiting time shorter. The sessions were not what I expected, even though I wasn't entirely sure what to expect. Mostly we sat in silence. Everything apparently had to come from me. I did not know where or how to start. I had become so used to keeping all my feelings locked away it was very difficult to open up. I dreaded going to the sessions as there was no prompting, no clues on what to say or anything. It felt very intense and awkward.

My mood dropped even lower and I found it hard to even do everyday tasks such as cleaning, or even getting ready in the morning. I had little energy and woke up early every day around 3 o'clock time and struggled to go back to sleep. I cried a lot and felt very anxious. My bingeing and purging continued. I felt weighted down with a dark heaviness, like a black shroud covering me. I found little joy in anything anymore. I had a lot of morbid thoughts about death and suicide and fantasised every day about killing myself. I felt utterly worthless and full of guilt. My GP was concerned about me and arranged for me to see a psychiatrist.

One thing that seemed to relieve my symptoms a little was going for a drive in the evening. Michael would take me out in the car for a drive in the country or just around the city. Somehow this made me feel a little better and not as full of despair. My thoughts in the car started to become morbid as I kept thinking about ending my life by jumping out of the car whilst we were travelling. I obsessed over this thought and found myself willing myself to do it, it would be the end, the end of this suffering. Each time we went out I had this thought screaming at me loudly in my head.

I did not want to see anyone and cut myself off aside from my close family.

My appointment came through to see the psychiatrist, it was at Woodside Grange Hospital. This was an old mental hospital in

Narborough, Leicester. It was where my aunty had stayed many years ago and I had visited as a child. Michael went with me as he was worried about the state I had got into. I was sobbing uncontrollably a lot of the time. I didn't know why I was crying, just that I felt utterly depressed. I waited to see the doctor inside the old building. It was very creepy inside with long shadowy corridors and old worn rooms. It was like something out of a horror film that I used to love watching. I could hardly speak to the doctor through my tears. They decided straight away that I was to be admitted.

I was taken onto a ward and sat in the lounge area with Michael. I felt scared at being left there as there was a lot of activity in the room with some patients behaving oddly and some were loud. Part of me wanted to stay as well as it felt safer to be locked away than to be outside in the world. I had not been coping very well at all.

I was given a bed in a dormitory and Michael left me to go home and fetch some of my things, clothes and toiletries. A nurse spoke to me whom was admitting me to the ward. I recognised her from school, she had been in my class. When I mentioned this to her she didn't seem to recognise me and I felt stupid for mentioning it. She probably thought I was crazy and part of my illness. I stayed in my bedroom area until Michael returned, then after a short while he left to go home. I felt alone and scared in that hospital. One lady spoke to me and she seemed as high as a kite, she told me she was manic. She didn't stop talking and buzzing around the place.

I was put on new medication after seeing the doctor. I had been taking some form of anti-depressant since it all began when I was fifteen. The shame of it. I wanted to be normal. I was given a tranquilliser as well which helped calm the crying down and I felt sleepy a lot of the time. The days were a blur of lying around on my bed or pacing up and down the ward. There was nothing to do and time went very slow. My family visited and this upset me as I felt so ashamed to be in this situation yet again. What was wrong with me? I had heard the label "Endogenous Depression" and "Chronic Depression" used by the professional staff.

After a couple of weeks, I felt a bit improved and less anxious and wanted to go home. They let me be discharged and I was an out patient.

Back at home I spent a lot of time on my own again, but felt better than I had before. My mood was brighter and I didn't feel sick with anxiety as I had before, nor had thoughts of ending my life. I saw my family and Michael's family and tried to keep occupied. I took up cross stitch and spent many hours sewing different designs. It was very therapeutic.

Michael's mental health had suffered during this time as he had been worrying about me and about surviving financially. I felt even more guilty.

The weeks went by and I went downhill again, my mood worsened. I went back to see my GP and asked to be readmitted. This time my mum took me to hospital. My relationship with Michael had become very fraught and he was struggling to cope with our situation.

I befriended two people in hospital this time, a lady called Joy, who only stayed for one night and an older lady called Edna. It turned out that Edna lived near to me. I kept in touch with Joy. Edna took me under her wing. She was very sweet. I also got to know a lad, my sort of age, in his twenties a little as well. It was close to Christmas and one day I left the ward to go Christmas shopping as I had done nothing and had bought nobody any presents. It felt surreal leaving the ward to do this and my heart pounded as I walked around the city centre. I felt really upset as well as my relationship seemed to be deteriorating further. I went home for Christmas and spent some time apart from

Michael. I felt as though his family were angry with me and blamed me for making him unhappy.

I returned back to Woodside Grange for a short time after Christmas before I was discharged.

I continued to spend a lot of time doing my cross stitch as found it really helped me to occupy my mind.

It improved between Michael and I gradually.

After a few months of recovery I decided to try some voluntary work to start building up my confidence again and meeting new people. I got a placement at major charity shop working in one of their shops in town. I spent most of my time on my shifts working behind the scenes, sorting and pricing clothes and household goods that were donated. It was interesting as you never knew what you would come across and the people were nice and friendly. Sometimes I would do a shift in the shop on the till. One day, two men came in and asked me for something. I didn't have what they wanted and one of them called me a fat cow on his way out. This really hurt me and knocked my confidence somewhat for a while. At this point in time, I wasn't hugely overweight, just slightly.

I worked in the charity shop for many months, gradually gaining more confidence in their safe environment. I felt better about myself than I had for a long time. I felt very insecure within though, deep down, and I really wanted Michael and I to get married. We didn't have much money between us with my not working for quite some time, but we planned a wedding on our tight budget with help from our parents.

CHAPTER FOURTEEN
SELF HELP

My outpatient appointments at a local psychiatric Hospital became less frequent. I was wanting to be free from that world again as I felt such a great amount of shame attached to it, it made me feel like I was less of a person and that I could not cope. I just wanted to be normal and be seen as normal. Somewhere in my mind I longed to be successful, as that would be as far removed from what I considered myself to be as possible. Successful in a career, working my way up the ladder to the top or my own business as I had seen my dad achieve for years. I had visions of myself in a suit and making important decisions and making a difference in the world. Travelling with my work appealed also and had a glamorous image.

Even though I was coping outwardly a lot better than a few months earlier, I still had a lot of inner turmoil to contend with. Each day, each hour, many of the minutes, it was relentless. My voices telling me I was not good enough, I was a failure, I was not worthy. It exhausted me to always be fighting these thoughts. I read many, many self help books on Bulimia, Depression, Anxiety and personal development books hoping for my answer. I took great interest in anything linked with psychology and mental health to help me with my struggles. I was determined to be happy and at peace. The thing I found most comforting and therefore helpful was reading about other people's experiences. I loved true stories where I could identify with the author, it stopped me from feeling quite as alone and as much as a weirdo as I did. Maybe one day I would write my own, I had always wanted to become an author with my love of creative writing. I did not write as much these days but still loved to read. I decided it would be a good idea to write again and I fancied writing to penpals, so I joined a universal penpal club. Before long, I had penpals from all around the world and we were regularly exchanging letters. It was good, as it gave me something positive to focus on.

Our wedding day was organised and we even managed to budget for a short honeymoon in Paris. We both loved Paris and had visited the city when we had first met. We kept it to a small occasion with family and close friends only invited. Not only were we on a tight budget with me not earning but I didn't want too much fuss.

August 17th came around and it turned out to be the hottest day of the year. I loved Michael but I don't think I was in love with him and I don't think he was with me. We were both quite lost souls in a way and we felt as though we needed one another. This may have been wrong and not enough of a reason to marry but it was for me. We both knew of our struggles individually and in our relationship. We had been for some relationship counselling a while back which had helped.

It was a wonderful special day and I did feel happy. I wore a pale pink suit, a skirt with a matching short sleeved jacket and white shoes and handbag to match the trim on my suit. I knew my exact weight and even though it wasn't the weight I had hoped for on my wedding day, I felt okay and not too fat. Michael wore his navy suit. We chose a register office to get married in as neither of us was religious and it was simpler. As we came out of the building I loved the confetti being thrown at us, it was like out of a film. Afterwards we went to a nearby venue for a champagne toast and the wedding cake was cut. It did feel magical. It was very hot and sunny outside, so when people had started to leave, we walked to our next venue. Just the close family attended a special meal at one of the best restaurants in the city centre. We took random photo shots on the walk to the hotel which captured the moment beautifully. There was more champagne at the meal, and even though the food was delicious, I was so excited I could hardly eat, I lost my appetite. That night we stayed at the hotel, my dad had treated us. It was a beautiful room, but there was very little romance. I remember thinking that a wedding night was not meant to be this way and then brushed it aside. We went home the following day after a lovely breakfast. We poured over the wedding cards and gifts, feeling very lucky and spoilt in a good way. Later on, we met with some of my family and went out for a pub drink, the weather still sunny.

Our honeymoon in Paris lasted for four days, three nights. We walked miles and saw a lot of the sights we wanted to see and some revisited from last time. We had just got married but I felt we were more like brother and sister or friends. We enjoyed our trip all the same.

A few months later, I saw my GP and I said that I felt like trying to find work again, she agreed. The search began again, job applications galore and CV's sent off. I went from job to job again for a while. I didn't know what I wanted when it came to it, I was only truly qualified to be a chef but did not want to do that again. I worked in a herbal clinic for two weeks but hated that. Then I went to work in an accountants office, I felt very out of my depth and it soon showed and they asked me to leave in the end. I did some more retail work which I managed okay and enjoyed customer service even though I was constantly fighting anxiety and critical thoughts.

I thought I might enjoy working in travel and went along to a mass interview for a travel company. I had to sit and listen to a presentation in a large room before we were individually called in for interviews. I was one of the last to be called in and by this stage I was a bag of nerves. I made my excuses to a member of staff and hurried out of the building as fast as I could. I burst into tears and felt so frustrated with myself as I usually managed to pull off a good interview at least. My dad knew the owner of the business and he kindly arranged for me to have a separate interview back at one of the branches. This went okay but I did not get the job, hardly surprising after my first performance.

The months slipped by. I was very disillusioned with my still not coping very well in the workplace. I tried working back at my old optician's firm at a different branch, but had got myself into such a state internally again. I worried myself sick before I went and by the time I arrived I went to pieces and kept crying, I had to go home. I applied to another optician's and got an interview, which always pleased me. It was the start of the summer and we were about to go away to Cornwall on holiday for a fortnight. I had to ring whilst we were away to find out whether I was offered the job or not. Cornwall was beautiful as always, I had spent many holidays there as a child growing up. Towards the end of the holiday I rang the optician's, I was thrilled when they offered me the job to start the following week. Goodness knows what Michael must have thought, here we go again no doubt. I felt ashamed.

The optician's job lasted just a few days as I convinced I was no good at it and did not fit in. I kept crying and worrying the whole time. Dismayed, I went back to see my GP. She was very understanding and signed me back on the sick for a while again until I got myself sorted out.

It put more of a strain on my marriage again. I was not happy and neither was Michael deep down.

I read more books and went to some drop in groups for people with mental health problems. I really wanted to speak to people whom felt like me, if there were any. I found a couple of Eating Disorder groups to try out. I went to one on my own but never went back as I felt too ashamed even of that. I went to another a bit further afield in Melton Mowbray, Michael drove me there and came in with me. This was a better group for me and it was good to talk to people whom I felt understood. The leader was a recovered bulimic. I remember her saying that she went shopping daily so that there was never any food much in the house. I wondered if this was recovery. It made sense to do that and I would if it was just me living on my own. As it was, if we had any goodies in, such as sweets or cakes, I always asked Michael to lock them in his car so that I could not get them when I was desperate to binge. The compulsion was that strong. Mind you, this did not deter me, as I still bought food secretly or concocted things in the moment from raw ingredients. Once a binge took hold, that was it. I had often eaten frozen food or semi defrosted in a frenzy and had even resorted to picking scraps of food out of the bin. It was disgusting, I knew it and felt it but I still could not stop.

Michael and I went for some more counselling together at Relate as we came very close to splitting up. We had booked a holiday to Greece months before but our relationship had deteriorated and we decided not to go and lost our deposit. Relate did help again, but part of me knew we were just grasping at straws, clinging to one another in an unhealthy way. Each time I was the one to talk about us breaking up but when it came to it I begged us not to. It was a mess.

CHAPTER FIFTEEN
ANOTHER LIFE ON THE WAY

I was now in my late twenties, Michael and I were still together. My mum knew I was not happy but it seemed to me like a lot of couples were not, and this made me feel better. We went out a lot at weekends as we always had, I think this really helped to keep us together. We were both quite shy people, but I definitely had a more outgoing streak than he did and wanted to socialise more.

We had the internet and I spent quite a lot of my time online. Searching for help, my never ending mission to be happier. I joined a forum for other people with mental health issues and it was good to chat to other people that had a good idea of what this life was like. I also made a friend that lived locally, she was really nice and we met up. I also looked at a lot of Eating

Disorder websites and there was becoming a trend in "pro anorexia" sites. I found myself looking out of curiosity but did not like them as they triggered a lot of not so good feelings and thoughts. They were actually promoting the benefits of having anorexia, which on my gut level seemed very wrong but I was drawn to them all the same. They were sharing techniques on unhealthy habits such as how to avoid eating, and how to make yourself weigh heavier to deceive medical staff. There was also discussion about the voices and suicide. There was always that competitiveness in me, which I knew derived from not feeling good enough but it did drive me on, so there was a positive to it. One morning I woke up and sobbed. I said to Michael that I actually did not know how to eat anymore. I could not remember normal eating or what to eat. My addiction had distorted everything. Just eating something for breakfast could be enough to trigger a large binge. Every day I made myself refrain from bingeing for as long as possible, I was like a time bomb waiting to explode. I both hated it and still got some benefit from it. I didn't know how on earth I would ever break free from this cycle. It was helping me to avoid thinking about painful memories and helped me with my fears for the future. As I gave way to a binge, I almost went into a kind of haze, everything would be blotted out and I just focussed on the act. Purging became harder to achieve and it sent me into a big panic. If I could not throw up, I would get fat and that was my biggest fear of all. I'd become very adept at making myself sick, but now as I rammed my fingers down my throat, not much would come back up. I tried drinking lots of water which often helped but it still did not make much of a difference. It was very scary. I resigned myself to being stricter with my diet and researched more diets that I could find, all offering me weight loss and the dream of being happy.

I found that by going out of the house as much as possible

helped me, as a distraction, and by being around other people. It got to the point that I never wanted to be on my own for this reason and I panicked when I had to be alone. A binge would be inevitable followed by getting rid of it.

My weight stayed quite stable, fluctuating by only a few pounds but it had a massive grip on me and my self worth was measured by that figure on the scales.

I tried going back to work. I didn't fancy retail again and all of my other efforts in other jobs had failed so there was only catering that I knew. I felt so bad about being out of work all of the time and forced myself to get a job. I found a job in a nursery as the cook and this was a nice set up and I felt more at ease. It was a pleasant environment to work in with the children and babies and I got on okay with the girls that worked there. It was part time so not too challenging and I was finished after lunchtime each day. I felt much better going out and earning my own money rather than keep relying on sickness benefit.

My GP always told me not to be so hard on myself, but she did not feel the shame of it. At twenty seven, I had barely held down a full time job and the longest I had worked anywhere was just over a year, and that had felt near impossible. It did not do much for one's self esteem.

I managed to refrain from bingeing at work and was very pleased with myself about that. Working in the nursery also had another effect on me, I became broody.

Michael and I had said that we did not want children. I felt as though I could barely look after myself, never mind be responsible for another human being. Plus we barely had a sex life so it would be a challenge on that front. It seemed a simpler life choice.

As the weeks passed, my maternal instinct really kicked in and I knew that I really wanted a baby, despite any thoughts I'd had previously. Suddenly this overwhelming desire took me over and I felt it even more so at work. I found myself noticing all babies when I was out. I told Michael how I felt and after much discussion he agreed.

I also knew that what I had put my body through the past seven years with my eating disorder, and still was, that I had reduced my chances of being able to conceive. That upset me and it was a big incentive to stop my habits. They certainly dwindled as I thought more and more about getting pregnant.

Amazingly, I became pregnant almost straight away. I was overjoyed. I was bursting to share my news with family and friends. That was it, this was my reason to stop bingeing and look after myself better, at least until my baby had been born. And I did. It was easier than I thought, being terrified of harming the little person growing inside of me stopped my urges. I started to feel better than I had done for a long time. I had the usual tiredness at the beginning but otherwise I bloomed.

At work, I felt pressured by my boss and did not like the job anymore. So I looked for another job and found another one in a nursery as a cook. This was closer to home too so more convenient especially now I was pregnant. I felt guilty not telling them I was in the early stages of pregnancy when I started but I had to keep earning money now more than ever. Having a baby was expensive, but I was so excited at the thought of becoming a mum.

I worried a lot in my pregnancy, as I always did, old habits and all, especially at work. I was not bingeing but did overeat. I consoled myself with the thought that I could lose all of the weight once my baby was born. Considering I had such hang ups about my shape and a rigid control of my weight, I adapted to my changing shape very well. I loved my pregnancy and felt really special. It was such a relief not to be as obsessed about my food and weight as much and not spending as much time in the bathroom. We saved money too as I wasn't buying binge foods. I must have spent a small fortune on food over the years for it to be abused.

I had to tell them at the nursery after a few weeks and they were very understanding, which made me feel more guilty. I stopped carrying heavy trays of food and was generally looked after. As my growing bump emerged, the children at the nursery took an interest. There was one little boy in particular, he was so cute and he took a shine to me.

I went out and bought a really good pregnancy and baby book as I wanted to understand everything that was happening to my body over the nine months and about looking after a baby afterwards. I had no experience and had never even baby sat for anyone never mind changed a nappy.

We gradually purchased baby items and decorated the spare room and turned it into a nursery. I found out I was expecting a boy and we were thrilled. Choosing a boys name was more of a challenge and it was narrowed down to about three. Joseph became the favourite.

This had to be the happiest time ever of my life as I really bloomed and had something magical happening that would change our lives forever. For the first time in a very long time, I truly felt as though I had something to really look forward to. The future was bright.

Towards the end of my pregnancy I stopped working and really enjoyed the last few weeks. It was tiring and physically uncomfortable at times but I loved it. I was so looking forward to meeting our son. When it got really close to my due date in late January 1999, a new panic set in. I confided in my mum, that I felt like I wouldn't cope or know what to do. It's almost as though I wanted to change my mind, but obviously there was no way that could happen. I worried a lot.

My due date came and went. I had heard all of the old wives tales about bringing on labour and tried eating curry and walking up the very steep hill near to my house but nothing worked. One night, I started to have pains, which I guessed were contractions and a show. The pains continued for a few hours and we contacted the hospital. They asked us to come in. The pain was mostly in my back but on examination I was barely dilated and told to go home. At home I had a bath as suggested but was in agony and on all fours as the pain was all at the back. I felt as though I wasn't taken seriously. Eventually they waned, and the next day we went out to get some essentials. In the shop the contractions started again but kept coming and going for hours. I got into a state and the pain was wearing.

Later that day, the contractions got stronger and I was convinced the baby was going to appear any time. I went into hospital and they decided to induce me as I was still only three centimetres dilated. I was put into a bed, monitored and hooked up to a drip. I called my mum and told her I'd made a mistake and wanted it all to go away. Who was I to think I could be a good mum? Labour progressed and the lower pain was excruciating and it went on and on. All of a sudden, I was thrust a form to sign. My baby was in distress and I needed to have an emergency caesarean. We were both scared.

I was rushed off to theatre and the next thing I knew, Michael was dressed in a green overall and standing next to me and holding my hand. I was given an epidural, then moments later after much rummaging sensation, our son was born into the world. The doctor held up a little boy taken from my womb.

CHAPTER SIXTEEN
JOSEPH

At ten minutes to nine, on Saturday February 6th 1999, Joseph was born. The three of us were taken into a side room to rest and bond together for the first time for a few hours. It was hard to believe as I looked at my little boy for the first time, he was truly beautiful and perfect. His tiny little features and hands. Amazing. I still felt numb from the operation but so grateful that everything had turned out well and that Joseph was safe. We made a few phone calls to let our families know of our news. My mum was overjoyed and I heard the excitement in her voice, she said that I sounded like a young girl at the end of the phone. I wanted to do the very best for our son and wanted to breastfeed him. I was shown what to do by a midwife and after a few attempts I managed to get Joseph latched on and drinking my milk. We were moved to our own little room and once settled, Michael went home to get some sleep and get ready for our return home. For me, not one, but two new lives had been born. I was going to change for Joseph.

I felt very tired after a long slow labour and the caesarean, but I could not stop looking in amazement at the little bundle of gorgeousness next to me in his little hospital baby bed. He had dark hair and was quite red in appearance and a little screwed up like babies do. His little cry was surprisingly loud for a tiny little thing. He was just over seven pounds in weight. I fed him again throughout the night.

The next morning, Michael came to visit us. By now, I could feel everything again after the injection had worn off, it was very painful to move. He helped me to get to the bathroom and somehow shuffle myself into the bath. I was covered in dried blood and a dressing. I saw myself in a mirror and could not help but check out my shape and size. It did feel better to get clean though and I was encouraged to move carefully but to keep moving. We then had the task of changing Joseph's nappy for the first time, as the midwives had helped out during the night. There was going to be a lot of firsts.

Our families came to visit and some close friends and we were inundated with new baby cards and presents for Joseph. In between the visits, I suddenly had a lot of pain in my arm and chest and my breathing was difficult. I was whisked off for a scan, as they thought I may have a blood clot but thankfully all appeared to be okay.

We stayed in for a few days before we were allowed to go home. It felt daunting to go home, away from the support of the hospital and the staff. Joseph had his first journey in his little car seat. We arrived home and showed him his new home and his room. The nursery was painted sunshine yellow with a bright colourful animal border and matching curtains.

I felt really lost and had a panic attack. Michael called the doctor and our GP came out to see me. As I was breastfeeding, I was advised on my medication. I was determined to continue breast feeding, my son deserved to have the best I could provide for him. I already felt as though I'd let him down with the birth and how it turned out. I'd wanted a water birth and it to be as natural as possible.

As Michael was in a new job, he could only get one day off. My mum came over a lot to support me in the first few weeks, especially as I was recovering from my operation too. I got into a routine with Joseph and tried to rest when he did as much as possible. He slept in a little Moses basket next to our bed at night. I was feeding him on demand and quite a lot, but I was grateful for the chance to rest. I started to fill out a baby book with our first memories.

During late pregnancy, I'd found a lump in my breast, and now they called me for a scan to investigate. My mum came with me to the appointment and we were there for several hours, in between feeds. It turned out to be a harmless cyst.

I began to venture out and went for walks with Joseph in his pram once my six weeks check was done and my scar was healing well. I felt so much love for this little boy but I felt quite lonely as well. I did not have any friends with babies or young children, so I decided I wanted to meet some, for both of our sakes. I saw a poster in my doctors surgery for new mums and replied to the number. I met up with a lady called Shelley and her baby who lived quite close by and then we both joined a local mother and toddler group. It was daunting to begin with, but Joseph was only a couple of months old and slept through most of it. It gave me the opportunity to chat to other mums. We made other friends and went to more groups. I loved my new life as a mum. I felt much happier than I had ever done in my life.

I was not happy with the weight I now was and had hoped that I would have naturally lost more after the birth, so I embarked on a sensible diet as I was still breastfeeding. I had no desires to binge or throw up however and that amazed me. As more time passed, I began to think I was free of that forever. I hardly dared to believe it but it seemed to be a reality. Slowly I lost weight and this pleased me as I could fit back into some old clothes gradually, instead of having to wear baggy clothes or some maternity jeans.

We went out most days and developed a great social life. We made many friends and went to playgroups, baby gyms, and other mum's houses. In the summer we went on lots of day trips and picnics at parks, it was a wonderful new life. As Joseph grew, his character developed more and he was a happy little chap. I could tell he was going to be strong willed though.

I took to being a mum like a duck to water and felt secure feeling I was at last doing something with my life that was very worthwhile. Money was tight for us, but we agreed I could stay at home and be a full time mum as it was what I really wanted to do. I wanted to be the best mum I could and give Joseph everything and to nurture him. We managed to get away on holidays still and took so many photos to treasure.

At around ten months old, I felt a swift decline in my mood and saw my GP. She felt it was delayed post natal depression and I went back onto medication. Thank fully I improved as fast as I declined. I did not want those awful feelings to spoil my time with my baby.

We had a big party for Joseph's first birthday, as we didn't have a christening and wanted to celebrate with family and all of our new friends. I made him a novelty cake, a yellow duck, and knew it would be the first of many. I loved doing things for Joseph.

We reached all of the usual milestones, crawling, walking,

speaking and eating. It was an incredible journey. We took Joseph on his first holiday abroad to France. We wanted to take him to Disneyland Paris when he was two years old and we fitted in a trip to the city whilst there as well. I felt really thin on that holiday and it felt satisfying to fit into smaller clothes again. I ate rather strictly and would not allow myself many treats.

Deep down, I felt unhappy in my marriage. It was rearing its head again. It felt even more apparent as I had new found confidence through being a mum and our new set of friends.

Joseph started to be known as Joe sometimes. When the time came for Joe to start at nursery at the local school, I sobbed and was beside myself for the first week. He only went for a couple of hours most days but it felt like a huge loss. He settled in well though and made some new friends. I always felt isolated at the school whilst waiting in the playing ground with the other mums. Even though I joined in with conversations, I felt alone. It reminded me of how I had felt before in the past. I didn't like it.

I felt pressured in my marriage as I didn't feel very close to Michael now and was more irritated than anything. We were very different and the difference really showed now. I craved more excitement in my life and to feel passion which there was a lack of. It got harder as time went on and I reached the point where I could not bear him to be near me.

I was not feeling good about myself or my marriage. Slowly I began to turn back to familiar habits, with the occasional binges and purging. I shocked myself and was deeply disappointed as I thought this was a thing of the past. As addictive as it was, I was soon back to regular binges and purging cycles. If nothing else, it helped me to cope with my marriage.

One day, when Joe was playing in the lounge with his toys, I felt an overwhelming desire to binge. Making sure he was safe, I shut the stair gate behind me fixed in the lounge doorway. As

I could hear his playful little voice I savaged the contents of our kitchen cupboards, desperately shoving food down my throat. Such a relief. Feeling glimpses of guilt, I shoved more food into my mouth. Michael was in the garden and how could I do this to our little boy. What kind of a mother was I? After reaching a point of extreme fullness and discomfort I knew I had to rid myself of the calories. I couldn't go upstairs and so proceeded to throw up in the kitchen bin. I could still hear Joe and knew he was okay and safe. Then suddenly, Michael barged into the kitchen. I hadn't heard him come through the back door, he caught me in the act. I felt like a rabbit caught in headlights and he got angry and shouted at me. How could I do this when our son was playing next door? I know, how could I? I asked myself the very same question. I felt utterly ashamed of myself, and rushed upstairs to the bathroom. I finished throwing up, then cleaned myself up and went back downstairs.

Later on that day, I apologised to Michael and cried a lot when I looked at my beautiful son. I said I would get help again.

CHAPTER SEVENTEEN
TWO NEW LIVES

As I looked at my gorgeous little boy I knew that I could not do this to myself again and certainly not to him. I wanted to protect him and give him everything I had not had in life and this would not cut it.

It was all too familiar seeing my GP and asking for help yet again. I felt as though I ought to be able to sort all of this out on my own, I was an adult and now a mother. I'd already had lots of help from the NHS and felt somewhat greedy asking for more. But I did not know what else to do, as it felt too complicated to sort out by myself. The books had helped, but it felt like there was so much more to unravel.

Another referral later, and I was seeing a specialist at the local hospital in the Eating Disorders unit. I had a feeling of déjà vu.

The therapist was a nice lady and I was able to open up to her. It was recognised how much I struggled to let go of negative thoughts and events. I said to her that if I knew how to let go I would. I had tried all of the usual visualising about putting things in a box or cutting a tie but nothing seemed to shift.

After the second or third session she remarked that I hardly spoke about my marriage. It all came tumbling out, how deeply unhappy I was and the lie we were living. That day, I went home and told my husband the marriage was over.

Almost overnight, I stopped the food and eating rituals. I could not believe it. The shift in myself was dramatic. Michael was very upset and angry with me. I explained to him that it was the right thing to do for us both. We had come close several times before but this time it would be permanent for everybody's sake. I moved into the little box room which we just used for junk and borrowed a camp bed from a friend. Some of my family and friends were a bit judgemental about my decision I felt but it was not an easy one to make in the first place.

Living in the same house was difficult. We tried to keep things amicable for Joe's sake and we mostly achieved this. Not long afterwards, Michael was very upset one day and was in tears. I felt for him. I was not in love with him but I did not want to see him so distressed. I knew he had been for some counselling and I thought it was because of our break up. He was finding it hard to speak and from somewhere, I have no idea where, I guessed what the problem was. I asked him if he was gay. He said he was. It must have come from my subconscious self as I had never suspected that from him. He was never a very manly man and I often felt like it was me wearing the trousers so to speak, but I was shocked to the core.

As I turned over thought after thought and memory after memory in my mind, a lot of things started to make sense to me. He revealed some of his thoughts to me which hurt a lot but I also could see the strain he had been under. When I had been jealous when we dated he had been looking around, but not at women, at the men. It wasn't just my paranoia then. He had never said anything about it to anyone or done anything about it which must have been very hard to live that way too. We both had our secrets. We agreed that Joe was too young to understand and we would explain to him when he was older.

Even though breaking up felt freeing, I also felt very vulnerable as my need to be with someone came back with a vengeance. The thought of being on my own was too much too bear and I felt so unloved.

I had been chatting to a lady online in one of the Eating Disorder forums about her son who was anorexic. I suggested that I could meet him as they lived locally, to see if I could help. I also secretly wondered what he was like. I went to meet him at his home, he was eleven years younger than me. His name was Drew.

He was in recovery apparently but he still was very thin. We talked and I could tell straight away that we shared a real connection. Both with similar fears and beliefs about the world. I arranged to see him again.

In my mind, I began to fantasise about him being my boyfriend possibly. We saw each other more and romance blossomed, and I certainly helped it on its way. He knew of my situation and he lived with his dad.

Michael and I lived under that same roof for about six months until it became too frustrating. He found out that I was seeing Drew, and was really angry at me. He had begun to visit gay bars in town so I did not know how he could be so angry with me. It was a two way street. It felt as though when we were happy once, we were not really, as it was all a big lie.

The house was up for sale and in the end, I moved out with Joe to a rented house whilst Michael stayed in the house until the sale went through. Our beautiful cat, Daisy, stayed with Michael. We found a nice house locally and we lived next door to one of our close friends, with another in the same street. It was a wonderful support network. There had been a lot to sort out at once, unpacking everything, arranging benefits, and getting Joe settled and selling our house. I think some of the emotions got pushed down as at times as they were too painful and too much to deal with at once. I only binged and purged from time to time, nothing like it was.

I felt a freedom that I had not ever felt, a big release and I started to enjoy it. At the same time however, the relationship with Drew continued but it became obvious that he was not truly in recovery and behaved very oddly a lot of the time. He withdrew a lot from seeing me which really hurt. I felt very unlovable. His mum could not understand why I was with him as she knew how entrenched he was in his own beliefs. I really felt connected to him and loved him. Even though it was also very painful as he was not free to love me truly. His eating disorder was still number one.

Joe settled in and seemed very happy considering he had his parents break up. He was three years old and had lots of love. Michael saw him regularly so it gave me some free time. I started to go out a bit to nightclubs and bars, living the life I never had in my teens. We had filed for divorce and we went for a few sessions in mediation. They were very uncomfortable sessions but we managed to make important decisions about custody without the need to go to court. It was the last thing either of us wanted.

Drew declared that he couldn't be in a relationship with me as he was too busy with his studies, he was doing a law degree. Really I knew this was more about his illness than anything else as he was in complete denial about it. I was heartbroken. I wanted to save him and so we live happily ever after with Joe.

I reacted by going out more and drinking and I had two one night stands, something I thought I would never do. I even had a really scary experience, when one night I went out in Nottingham with people that I did not know very well, and ended up getting my drink spiked. I collapsed in a nightclub toilet and came around several hours later in an office for the staff. I shocked myself, but I felt a desperate need to be loved and wanted. It hurt so badly. I think I was feeling more than I was used to as I was not pushing so many emotions and thoughts down with food. There was a big hole inside of me, a dark emptiness that needed to be filled with something to take away my pain. Food and purging filled it before, now there was nothing.

I could not be without Drew and we remained as friends. It was very hard. I wanted more.

Around the time that our house sold, Joe was due to start at school full-time. I also had to find somewhere else for us to live. There was a lot to juggle at once. I only viewed a few houses before I found something ideal for Joe and I, well as close to ideal as I would get on my tight budget. It was in the same area as there was no way I was going to disrupt his friendships he had made, he'd already had enough change in his little life. I remembered all too well how hard that was for me as well.

CHAPTER EIGHTEEN
ALL AT ONCE

The divorce proceedings were going through, and every now and then I would hear from my solicitor. It didn't matter how long it took, I was just relieved the break had been made and that we were both moving forward at last with our lives. A lot had happened in a short space of time and on reflection it surprised me how far I had come.

My offer was accepted on the new house, it was a two bedroom maisonette with a garden so that Joe could play outside. I gave notice on our rented house and got Joe settled in at school.

Drew was still in the picture but I spent much time crying and feeling rejected at his sometimes unkind behaviour. I made excuses as I knew it wasn't the true him but the anorexia and its evil grip. I was still putting up with it, that was more bearable than letting go.

Our house had sold and the sale went through quickly on our maisonette. I had bagged us a bargain. It needed a lot of work doing to it but I had some money leftover to take care of that. I couldn't wait to turn it into our home, for Joe and I. A fresh start.

I loved having friends and family over for dinner parties and get togethers, having our own space was fabulous. I soon got used to the different lifestyle. Joe's room was decorated first and we recorded his height on his bedroom door for fun. He was such a sweet and bright little child, I was so lucky to have him.

Now Joe was at school I began to look for work. It had been quite a while and part of me half expected me to fall apart again, but I didn't this time. I did not apply for many as now I had to fit work around school hours and they were hard to come by. By luck, a job came up as a merchandiser, locally and it was flexible working hours. I went for the interview and was over the moon when they explained that I could go in and do the hours at any time of the day or night. It was in a large twenty four hour supermarket working on a concession. I was elated when I got the job and this time I committed to it.

Our home gradually got revamped, we had great friends, Joe was happy and settled and I felt proud. It was a juggling act, this single mum life but I had no regrets whatsoever, I felt liberated to have broken free of my other unhappy life.

After a while my bulimic behaviour would creep in, at stressful times, but it was short lived each time. I'd have a blip, binge and vomit a few times then get myself back on track. It was manageable. I could go for several months of being completely free of it then engage in it for a short time. I recognised that I still had a lot of inner conflict, it was never ending. All of the years I had spent engrossed in self help books , always trying to change myself and move forward, it must have made a difference, but

I wasn't there yet. Believing I could one day be successful had always kept me going through my darkest days.

CHAPTER NINETEEN
MORE THERAPY

Our divorce came through. I even received a greetings card to congratulate me. It didn't really feel any different but I was pleased it was complete.

Drew and I had become closer again but I hardly saw him, it was a tortuous relationship but I could not seem to bring myself to end it. I was always hoping he would choose to recover and we could be happy.

I stuck to my job, I was often feeling upset inside, but I kept going each day. After time I felt bored and longed for more challenging work that would stretch my mind. I knew what I was like though and I needed stability. It was the longest I had ever stayed in a job, a new record set for myself.

I wanted to sort the rest of the "stuff" inside of me. There was much going on as I was always feeling my emotions triggered. I put my name down to see a private counsellor. I got to see someone quickly and I formed a trusted bond with the lady therapist very soon. I could really talk to her and I felt as though she really heard me and understood. This was amazing to feel, as I had never experienced this before. She really got me. We talked about a lot of my experiences with my family of when I was younger and as time went on, I felt as though I came to terms with a lot that had happened and made sense of many experiences in my mind. It was a relief to feel so understood. She was incredible and it helped me so much. I knew that I would always be very grateful to this special person.

Part of my healing was to speak to my family about aspects of the past and explain how I felt from my perspective. I was given new tools to use to help me cope. It was very hard work as each week I would leave having opened up old wounds and then I would have to cope for another week until my next session. I'd just be about getting over my distress when I'd be at my next appointment and it happened all over again. I sobbed almost every day for two years, sometimes crying for hours at a time. It seemed as though the tears would never dry up. I read more books that were recommended to me about reparenting and gradually old hurts were examined and put to rest. I learnt to have more compassion for myself and used old baby photographs to console myself with and sooth that young girl that had hurt so much.

I wrote a lot about my feelings and I felt continually rejected by most people. Everyone seemed caught up in their own world and had their own families. I felt uninteresting and unnoticed, no one wanted me really except my own son and he was seven. Towards the end of the two years of therapy I felt as though some old ghosts had been extinguished and I had a healthier relationship with my family and with myself. I talked about my relationship with Drew and why I was allowing myself to be so hurt continually. This then gave me the strength to finally let go, I was trying to save him and he didn't want to be saved. Part of it was me trying to save me. I was heartbroken but knew it was very unhealthy to keep that attachment alive.

At the end of the two years I did not want the counselling sessions to end as I knew there was still unresolved issues inside of me. My time was up at the counselling centre and she thought I had everything that I now needed. I was very inspired by how much this lady had helped me with such deep rooted and stubborn issues and I felt a deep desire that I wanted to do this for others as I knew how much difference it had made to me. Powerful stuff. She advised me against it when I brought it up for various reasons and I let that idea go for a while. We had our last session and I said goodbye.

Soon afterwards, I saw my GP and told her of the change that had taken place, she was very pleased for me. I said that I knew there were still unresolved issues for me and could I be referred for something else, I asked about CBT. She was happy to refer me.

My love hate relationship with food and my body continued, mostly staying away from my bulimic habits still and I kept my weight at a healthy level by counting calories, still rather obsessively, but I was in a much better place with it than before. I especially hated my stomach and as I had lost almost six stones, with a stone or so now gained, I had lose skin which hung in a small flap. It looked unsightly and I decided I wanted it gone. I began to research plastic surgeons and the treatments available. I soon had a proper bee in my bonnet about getting a tummy tuck, as my mum had always said, once I had made up my mind about something, that was it, I was like a dog with a bone. She was right. When I had an idea, there would be no stopping me! I chuckled to myself as I imagined myself with a new stomach, that would be amazing. I could see it now.

I asked for another referral through my GP to see a plastic surgeon. I had to see a psychiatrist first, oh joy I thought to myself. He had a cold manner and refused me to have the surgery as it was not severe enough and he felt it was more of a psychological problem. I was angry. Would I always be judged on my past? I had lost six stones, which at five foot was not a small amount on my frame and had loose surplus skin that no amount of exercise would shift. I liked and valued myself enough these days to care, which was a major improvement as to how I had felt about myself for most of my life. Hell, I was determined, and got myself an appointment with a private surgeon after more research. Financially I had no savings but found I could get a small remortgage and was going to fund it that way. Where there's a will there's a way. Always.

I had an assessment with a CBT specialist and he thought that CBT therapy would help me with my remaining issues with self esteem. I was put onto the next group course due to start in a few weeks, I was very pleased. I knew that I would do what it took to feel happy.

I saw the surgeon a second time and he marked my abdomen with a marker to show me where I would be cut and explained the procedure, I was having a mini tummy tuck as I didn't have enough skin for a full one. To me, this was an important step in my growing self esteem, to have a flatter stomach. I'd worked hard to change the inside. A date was arranged for my surgery and I would stay in overnight. Photos were taken of me and then others would be taken afterwards to show me the difference.

I didn't tell Joe what I was having done as I didn't want him to worry and he wouldn't understand. I just said mummy was having something done to her stomach as he knew how much pain I got with my ongoing IBS. He stayed overnight with one of my friends and she took him to school for me whilst I went into hospital and the other night with his dad. The night before I stayed with my parents and they took me out for a meal, I was so excited. I don't think they could truly understand why I wanted the operation done but supported my decision. The private hospital was so different to being in an NHS hospital. I felt very cared about and rather sadly, I really enjoyed my stay. The op was successful and I was bandaged up afterwards and a bit swollen so it would be a while before I saw the true results. As I lay resting afterwards in bed, I was thinking about all of the clothes I could now wear and how different I would feel. Gone were the days when I would keep comparing myself to other women and crying at pictures of models in magazines feeling fat and ugly.

My parents came into visit me and brought Joe with them, my dad made a lovely card for me.

CHAPTER TWENTY

BECOMING ME

I nursed myself but the recovery was fast from the mini tummy tuck and I only had to take two weeks off of work. I was excited to return for my check up and the swelling had reduced a lot. Another photo was taken of me and I was discharged. I did feel like a new woman and was very pleased with the results. There was a definite improvement and when I saw the photos it was remarkable to compare them. I looked different in clothes and felt a lot more confident in what I wore. I admired my new flatter stomach in the mirror every time I passed by a mirror, it made me happy so I knew it was the right decision.

I then started to think about meeting someone and embarked on the world of internet dating, as being a single mum, it was the easiest option for me. I even found a website for single parents and quickly I was hooked. It was fun chatting to men online and I soon got my first date. I was very nervous as I hadn't been on many dates before with different people, but I need not of worried. I felt really confident when it came to the actual date but was dismayed as the guy looked rather different than his online profile photo, I wasn't even sure it was him. I brought the date to a quick end and before he left he produced a bunch of flowers and chocolates for me. I felt relieved when he'd left and still unsure of his identity. I did not want the flowers or chocolates and gave them away to a neighbour. I did not let this experience deter me, and that night I logged back onto the dating site. I chatted to a few men but soon lined up a date with another guy. He seemed lovely and we arranged to meet. There was a drawback though as he lived miles away, up north. I decide to give it a try though, as nothing ventured, nothing gained. We got on really well and despite the distance between us we agreed to meet again. It went on for a few weeks until it fizzled out. We were not so compatible after all.

The CBT course had started and the group setting was okay. I spoke up more than I would have done in the past and I went out and bought the book they recommended. Each week we were given a lot of homework, but it was brilliant and made so much sense to me. Learning how to challenge and change your thoughts to change your behaviour. One of my challenges one week, was to go out without make up on as this is something I never did usually. I chose a day when I went to the gym and felt pleased when I managed it, but hated it at the time. Wearing make up made me feel much better and I liked to make the most of myself. I understood though that I had to feel good within as well though for true confidence. This was still a work in progress. We each had what was called a "bottom line", the ultimate belief we had about ourselves and what we thought others thought. Mine was "I am invisible".

Joe and I still enjoyed a good social life. He had made some close friends at school and I was friends with some of the mums. I never liked doing the school run though as felt the odd one out in the playground. I had never been the type of mum to be cooing over other mums babies or talking about potty training. I focussed on seeing Joe's little face when he came out of the classroom and asking him about his day. As he developed, I could see he was going to have a sensitive streak but he was so bright at school and his teachers spoke so highly of him. He was always keen to learn and began to get bored with the work set for him. I asked if he could have more challenging work set for him but it wasn't possible apparently. Not very encouraging I thought so we did what we could at home to nurture him and my brother was great at doing maths work with him.

I went on many first dates and did get rather obsessed about finding the right person. Whilst it was fun, I had some funny experiences and told myself that by the time I had finished I would be able to write a book.

Through the CBT I gained a lot of new confidence, it was an excellent help and really added onto the work I had done in my counselling. I learnt to speak up for myself more too and gradually my daily IBS pain subsided which felt like a small miracle after suffering for years. It was obviously triggered by my bottled up feelings that were not being expressed.

I met a fabulous guy online and I really fell for him, Jake. He was from Birmingham and recently separated and had the sweetest two daughters, I loved them. Things moved quickly and before I knew it we arranged to go on holiday together after our second date! Talk about impulsive. Strangely at the same time Drew got back in touch with me. This really threw me, I had said when we split to get back in touch with me if he ever decided to choose to recover. I heard him saying the words to me on the phone that I had longed to hear for the four and a half years we had been together. He had finished studying and had a job in law now. I was amazed as I didn't think he would get a job with the state of his health. He said he was changing his eating habits now too. We talked and I felt very torn. I told him that I had met someone else and was happy.

I went away with Jake on our holiday to Prague. I was also thinking about Drew whilst I was there and felt very confused. One day we went for a couples massage, and it made me cry which I tried to hide. I was thinking about Drew and all we had gone through. Then I thought about the pain it had caused and did I really want to risk that again, this with Jake, felt like it could be the start of something special. I shrugged off old memories and chose to enjoy my time with Jake. We had a blast and one of those days remains to be one of the best days of my life. We laughed from morning until night. The day was fuelled by plenty of wine drinking and eating. We did some sight seeing, then had a boozy lunch sitting outside in one of the grand squares. It was amazing scenery. Affected by the wine at lunchtime, I suggested we go on a horse and cart ride around the city. I could not stop laughing, I was in hysterics. Jake said afterwards that he could not keep up with me. Later on there was a big thunderstorm and the heavens opened. We found shelter in a bar and our drinking continued for several hours as the storm did. We were very loved up too and it felt wonderful, I felt so happy. The rain never let up and by early evening we searched for a restaurant to dine at, all of the drinking had made us hungry. We stumbled across the most beautiful restaurant, which was full except from a table outside but under cover. It was very atmospheric sitting outside with the rain pouring down and foreign music playing. We shared a bottle of red wine with our meal and again I got the giggles. The next thing I knew, I had stood up and pulled Jake to his feet and we danced undercover to the live music in front of everyone. We were applauded at the end and I did a mock courtesy to the crowd. Oh what fun!

As we left the restaurant in the rain, we both carried on laughing. I felt so alive. We were taking silly photos all day too and sharing private jokes. I got carried away with my joking about and went up to a random family in the street, they were dressed in raincoats. I got Jake to take a photo of me with them, they must have wondered what was going on. It was fun to be daft and carefree.

This happiness was short lived though. I had told Jake about Drew and him contacting me again and I knew he was upset. Then he began to talk about moving nearer to Leicester and part of me panicked as it felt it was moving so fast, I didn't feel ready for that yet. I asked him for some space and he took it badly. He refused to answer any of my texts or calls and eventually I got him to speak to me again. He came over to see me and I cooked us a meal. He said he could not go back to how it was, I knew he was finding it hard to trust as well as his wife had been unfaithful. That was it, it was over. It broke my heart as he would not change his mind, I only wanted it to slow down.

My way of dealing with this, as well as a binge or two, was to get straight back on the dating site. That way I did not have to think about the pain. Old habits.

CHAPTER TWENTY ONE
ANOTHER OBSESSION

Dating, in between work and looking after Joe, became all consuming. I tried different websites, after the chore of filling out my profile each time, it was fun to start chatting to men again. I set about making it my mission to find Mr. Right. Dating had given me a lot more confidence too and the fears I had held for years about relationships had vanished. I stayed up until the early hours most evenings chatting to people unless I was on a date. I was very determined, like the dog with a bone again.

Through all of the therapy I had been through and the changes that I had made, transformation really, the desire to help others grew. I looked into some training with a view to making a career change as Joe was getting older now and not quite as dependant on me. I embarked on several short courses and loved them all.

An introduction to counselling I loved and came away with a certificate. I also did Assertiveness training, Stress management, Person Centred Recovery, and Life Coaching. I felt in my element, and knew this path was right for me.

As well as online dating, I tried Speed Dating a few times. I met someone through this and we had a year long relationship. It had a lot of rocky patches as I did find it very hard to trust. Plus it meant introducing someone new to Joe again which really concerned me. After more rough patches, it just was not feeling right and I ended it for good. I found out by chance afterwards that he had been a cheat to his last partner and I had felt suspicious for good reason. It wasn't just my insecurity.

I began to look for a new job with my new skills. I had been merchandising for four and a half years, a record for me. There had also been a really horrible incident at work which pushed me into wanting to leave. An employee at work had sexually assaulted me in the store, in broad day light, he had put his hand down my trousers as I was leaning over to do my job. After reporting him, I was off for several weeks with stress and he was investigated. He kept his job and I had to return to the workplace. He broke the rules a few times about keeping his distance from me, I couldn't believe him. It was all very traumatic and for some reason I kept seeing him out of work also. It was uncanny and one day I shouted at him in the street to leave me alone. I was pleased to leave my job in the end as it was never the same again.

I got a job with a charity, supporting people with disabilities. Very different to anything I had done before, but it really appealed to me. I soon got into it and loved it, it was very rewarding and a privilege to work with these people. I was part of a team providing group settings to improve social inclusion and raise self esteem. We were like a big family and had some great times.

Joe got used to the after school club for a couple of days a week before he was old enough to have a key and let himself in after school. I trusted him and was proud of the sensible young man he was becoming.

I continued dating, as I still really wanted to be in a relationship. I felt it would complete me. When Joe was little, I knew I was trying to recreate that family unit I longed for, but not that anymore. I met someone else, and we became a couple quite soon. He was a heavy drinker it turned out and I found I started to drink more too. He also had a young son, and through what had happened to the boy's mum, he was very unruly. Whilst I felt for him, and it wasn't his fault, he was also very demanding and wanted attention constantly. He was mean to Joe as well at times and it caused problems. I really loved him but eventually it got too difficult. We never had time on our own and I was sick of the late night drinking and the chaos he lived in. We'd had a few breaks away as a family over the fifteen months and they had been anything but a holiday. I felt very guilty at what I had put Joe through, it was also very hard being a single mum. We had very different ideas about parenting and I called it off. I actually stopped dating for a while, after a few more first dates, it was very hard to meet the right person.

I threw myself into my work and I wanted to progress. The years of not feeling confident in the workplace had passed by and I had years of suppressed ambition inside of me. It had been immensely frustrating knowing I was capable of much more but not coping with more. I took on extra roles and was soon running an arts group each week. Then came an extra role in setting up a new group. I was working near enough full time and it was great for us to have more money. Then a job came up at work to become a group facilitator for the young persons services and I went after it. I knew I had given a great interview and was thrilled when I was offered the job. It was really sad to leave my old group but I knew I had more to offer.

Joe had started at high school and was issued his own front door key. He was growing up fast and was getting on very well.

The new job was challenging and I had a few wobbles but overall I coped well, considering how I had spent the majority of my life. I had more training, as part of my role was advocacy to young people in respite care. I was managing a team of people in my new groups and had to get used to presenting to the groups. My confidence grew further. I still had some wobbles inside, but that's all they were, nothing major. I felt proud of myself for the first time in my work, that was a special milestone for me. I missed working with my good friend Jem, whom had joined our group initially as a student. We had hit it off and soon became close friends. I loved her and we continued our friendship outside of work as we had done whilst working together. We were always meeting up and would chat for hours about all kinds of stuff, putting the world to rights.

I dated a little bit but nothing like I had been doing. I felt so much more fulfilled with my work. The emptiness I used to feel felt filled. I came across some journalling that I had written years before and was shocked to read the content. It did not seem like it was me I was reading about as I now felt so different. It saddened me to think I had once felt that way and for a long time but also a real sense of achievement of how far I had come.

Chapter Twenty Two
Old Triggers

Life felt the most stable it ever had. I was settled in work, Joe was doing better and better at school and we enjoyed holidays, trips and treats as I was earning a better wage.

My eating was very stable and my weight was too. I had gained some weight but I was okay with it as I recognised I had lessened the strict control I had once had. I still watched what I ate but was not continually counting calories which was so much more relaxing. I had been very stressed in my last relationship and had eaten more in that and had drank a lot more to match Pete's habits. It had helped me coped better with the chaos too, not the best method I realised but it was what I did at the time. I felt aching ambition inside of me that still wanted more. More responsibility and more of a challenge. I was getting bored in my job. Also there was the usual workplace politics that really frustrated me. I hated injustice of any kind.

I started on a job search once more, updating my CV which looked a lot more impressive these days. The jobs that I really wanted to apply for required either a degree or other qualifications I didn't have. I did not want to embark on intensive studying whilst working full time, as I wanted to still enjoy a social life. I continued to look for a more challenging job but one I was already qualified to do.

Eventually I found a new job. A shop manager for another charity. It was very different but it was a bookshop and I loved books. I cast my mind back to all of the reading I had done over the years. Mostly self development aside from a period of horrors in my teens. The thought of being surrounded by books thrilled me as there was always so much new to learn.

I was managing a team again, this time mostly volunteers. They were a lovely bunch and I formed a good working relationship with them all. It was great getting to meet new people as I only saw most of them for a few hours a week as they were all doing voluntary shifts. And the books, so many books, I loved it and was always excited when we had new donations or deliveries of the second hand books. Sometimes we had some real treasures come through the door and I found it fascinating. I think the whole process of sorting through thousands of books also appealed to my OCD nature.

Unknown to me at the interview, the shop was struggling to be financially viable. There would be quite a lot of pressure from management to increase the takings, even though the location was not doing the shop any favours. It was a lovely old shop on a quaint lane but not that much passing trade. They seemed very reluctant to new ideas which was hugely frustrating. They did however let me do one, and I embarked my family's help. My dad designed and made a book outfit and I convinced Joe to wear it to give out fliers to promote the shop in return for a small wage from my wage.

As time passed, I realised that I had made a less than desirable decision in taking on this job. There were so many restrictions and I found it so repressive. I worked full time but I was not allowed to leave the shop on my lunch break aside from fetching something to eat. I was continually pressured to make more profit for the shop and my boss was a bully. Some of the people that worked in the other shops seemed to enjoy gossiping and it became a very hostile working environment. Rumours went around that the shop was going to close and that people did nasty things to deliberately get others into trouble. I hated it and every day I felt like I was in a prison. I got depressed. I stood up for myself but my boss seemed to really dislike me and she made life difficult. It reminded me of my past bullying and I got very angry. My reaction to cope with it was to start bingeing and throwing up again. I was dismayed and very disappointed in myself after years of coping. I was not going to have it and saw my GP. She got me a referral back to the Eating Disorders unit. My mood spiralled further and my boss was really awkward with me taking time off to attend my outpatient appointments. I was so stressed. The shop did close but they opened up a new one in another town. I spent hours packing the shop up and giving it a thorough clean from top to bottom. I then helped to set up the new shop and worked long hours and came in on days off. It opened and I worked there for a few weeks. I hoped I could make it a fresh start.

Some of my closest friends were a great support during this time. It always made such a difference being able to talk to someone that you trusted and seemed to understand.

During this period we went away on a short holiday, me, Joe and my brother. We went to Paris on a coach trip. I really loved this amazing city and it drew me back time and time again. I cried whilst I was away and felt anxious but the physical distance from the work situation gave me some reprieve.

The therapist was brilliant and I had a short course of solution focussed therapy. It helped me to nip the eating behaviour in the bud and get back to a more normal eating pattern again. It got harder to be at work though and I knew I deserved better than this as the working conditions were still poor. In the end I got signed off with workplace stress and I took action against my managers for unfair behaviour.

Whilst I was off, I did a lot of thinking about what I was going to do.

CHAPTER TWENTY THREE
FOLLOWING MY DREAM

I didn't want to return to a bullying environment as it was obvious that nothing was going to change in their culture. I had meetings with the union which I had joined and HR of the charity and although I was heard that was going to be about it. I was offered the opportunity to move to another new shop that they were opening and to manage that but I was done, done with their ways and how they treated people.

A few months prior to this whilst I was frantically job searching, I had spotted a business idea generation course amongst the job adverts. I attended this for a few weeks and came away with a few ideas but nothing concrete and possibly more confused. Anyhow, I decided to take a look at this again. The idea of working for myself seemed very seductive as it would solve a lot of problems for me. The main being that I would not have to work in a toxic working environment again or having a boss making unfair demands on me. It also offered me the challenge I was craving and I still had my secret dream of being successful. I found links to another local business hub and investigated what was on offer. It sounded great, a business course to teach me all of the basics to get me started and also a business mentor. I decided to go for it and signed up, feeling excited at the prospect of a brand new start again in something entirely different. Re-inventing my life.

I took to the courses like a duck to water, I loved every moment and felt myself thriving. I found the leader in myself emerging again and it was a great feeling to be taking positive action.

With my mentor's help, I formulated an idea which became a plan, casting aside the other ideas that I had. I needed to be real right now as I was contemplating taking the leap into self employment, so whatever I did needed to be generating me an income for Joe and I to live on. Other ideas were going to take much longer to get up and running but this idea was doable immediately if I implemented what I needed to do.

I told my family and friends of my plans and they were encouraging. Only my dad really knew about the path I was going to take after his own journey for many years. I was very, very excited and began to do some mini research and buy the essential items that I would need to begin with my last months wages and borrowed a small amount from my dad. I was flooded with creative ideas and the possibilities were endless of what I could do, but I needed to focus on getting quick results. That meant gaining customers and sales.

Joe and I went out for the day, all the way on the train journey we were discussing a name for my new business. I was going to be selling jewellery, as I had always loved accessorising stemming from my goth days and wanted to help people at the same time. I had a keen eye for choosing items which were a little different to mainstream jewellery, with lots of ornate detail as I wanted the wearer to feel very special. A lot of thought went into how I would achieve this. I also knew I wanted to eventually grow it with people rather than purely selling online, as that did not motivate me. The thought of being able to offer a business opportunity to someone else inspired me hugely. There must be lots of people who had also found working for someone a real challenge. By the end of our journey I had a name for my business, Iridescence. This was chosen for a few reasons. I loved the name as it spoke for itself, sparkly array of colour and sounded sophisticated. I also chose a butterfly as a logo, as they have iridescent wings but it also signified the journey of change. From starting off in a tight cocoon, to flying freely, I could relate this to my own life. I may not be flying freely yet but its definitely where I was aiming for.

I went to the business hub once I had more essentials in place and asked for their support in registering my business formally. I felt anxious about this and it really helped to make the phone call to HMRC with them by my side. The joy I felt was incredible and I went home to tell Joe. I stood in my kitchen making a drink, then it really hit me of what I was making happen and I started screaming, whooping and punching the air! I felt amazing with a capital A. I really felt proud of myself for the first real time.

The first sale I had was to a lady on the business course with me and then another lady. That felt amazing, then I had a big launch party at home. I did well and friends and family supported me. My dad designed my logo and made me some point of sale.

Earning my money this way felt so different to getting a wage, so much more satisfying and getting the positive feedback was brilliant.

I looked at where I was going to find new customers. All the boring stuff had to be taken care of first and then I had to make a decision. My time on sick leave had come to an end, it was either find another job as I couldn't go back to the charity or make this business work. Sink or swim. That excited me massively in itself, that challenge. I took a deep breath, and quit my job, boy did that feel good! It was scary too but the excitement was more. I recognised this as my third big life change and I was sure going to embrace it.

I was learning new stuff thick and fast and it was a whirl but I absolutely loved it, I felt that this was going to be the making of me. I cried but it was tears of joy and I was so pleased with myself as I felt I was taking great strides to fulfil my big ambition. I had many obstacles in my way. No money saved up, single mum, not driving, but this seemed trivial when I compared it to what I had overcome in my life. Nothing was going to stop me – I was on fire!! The key was to see obstacles as challenges, relish them, and focus on how incredible it would feel to push past them and move forward. The focus was on what I wanted to achieve. My "why" was massive and my drive was matched. I felt that I had so much to prove to myself from all of my past years of unhappiness, shame, fear and failure. Joe was proud of me too which was really important to me to set him a great example of believing in yourself and going after what makes you happy in life.

My confidence increased triple fold and I worked like a crazy thing but I wanted to, I had a force of determination deep within me than had been tapped into and I was on one hell of a mission. I felt so fulfilled as my business progressed, all of my past seemed irrelevant somehow and I felt like a completely different person. For the first time ever I felt a strong sense of self respect. I felt very strong. I threw myself into the business world head first, networking and meeting lots and lots of other business people. I was so excited. I felt so alive. It had awakened a burning passion in me. For around the first six months, I would wake up early every morning bursting with enthusiasm to get going with the day and I would work until late at night most days and sometimes into the early hours. In that first eighteen months I averaged about eighty to ninety hours per week. Whilst I knew this was an unbalanced approach I also believed it was both what I needed to do to get things moving forward at the pace I wanted it to and I had this relentless driving force within me that did not want to stop for anything. I made a lot of sacrifices in that time, financially as I ploughed every penny, aside from for bills, back into the business to grow it. I had no partner to support me and yes it was very tough but I was hell bent on making it.

The first year it was just myself trading, with a little help sometimes with transport from my parents, mostly my mum. Aside from that I got around on public transport or taxis. Some of what I did may have been considered a bit crazy by some, but my mantra was always "where there's a will there's a way". Boy did this serve me!

I was trading everywhere I possibly could, organised events, workplaces, parties at peoples homes, more parties at mine, and I organised a couple of my own events too in two city centre bars. It was one long whirlwind of buying stock, displaying it, selling and doing it all over again. I put a lot of energy into building my brand and the style evolved as time went on and I found my niche within the vintage market. It made a lot of sense too, as much of the vintage jewellery is what I would have worn in my Gothic era. It certainly had an influence on my buying tastes and there was a demand for it.

After the twelve month mark, my first anniversary, I got my website and was delighted with the end result. I designed the look but someone built it for me. I had begun my pursuit with social media and that was taking off for me. I was on the case 24/7 or so it felt as there were notifications constantly on my phone or laptop. It was awesome! I started to get website sales with the amount of social media I was doing and they always felt so special, as if by magic, I'd have a sale notification in my inbox. I never got tired of that thrill. I built up my brand on four different social media platforms, mostly on Twitter and Facebook to begin with and gained some loyal customers. This meant a lot to me, as I was not selling a product that needed to be regularly replaced and it was tough in one aspect to keep finding new customers.

I had a big and very ambitious long term vision. So I set about formulating new strategies to make this happen to grow much further. I revisited my original idea about creating opportunities and focussed on that. I set up a party plan strategy where I would need to find a team of people to sell my products and they would earn a sales commission and I would earn the rest. The first person to join my business was a lovely lady called Karen. She loved the concept and the products and wanted to try her first taste at self employment. She loved it and we forged a great team.

That was it then, I was determined to find many other people to join my venture and grow this business huge. We had some teething troubles at the start, practicalities as there was a lot to organise and keep it running smoothly so I enlisted the help of two business advisors. I knew I needed a very firm foundation in order to achieve what I wanted to.

I continued to network and my name and brand was getting well known throughout Leicester, it took a lot of energy but it was a wildly exciting adventure and I was having the time of my life. On the rare occasion that I slowed down, and there honestly weren't many, I saw how much I had achieved and it spurred me on. I was getting further and further away from the person I used to be and that was the best feeling.

Joe was doing ever so well at school and as he matured he was showing signs of being a leader, an organiser himself. He seemed to be the one who organised the social activities with his friends mostly and I saw his confidence socially grow. He wasn't outgoing by nature but was quietly confident and very self assured. This is what I had really nurtured most of all in him, so he had good self esteem and confidence as that would take him a long way in life. I knew this all too well from not having had it for the best part of my life so far. He took an interest in business and maths especially and I tried to include him in my business, I paid him to do my book keeping each month. He also did a week of work experience with me from school and studied my business in a report he had to write for his business GCSE.

Throughout that year, I really focussed on growing my business and our team grew. It seemed a natural step and it was satisfying when there were enough of us to have regular team meetings. They were often in my home but sometimes we ventured out for a cream tea or elsewhere. I collaborated with models, bloggers and magazines. Writing a style advice column for a magazine and then getting featured in some national magazines was wildly exciting. Iridescence sponsored a national fashion week in Birmingham and I was nominated for several different business awards.

Each January it went very quiet after the frantically busy months of November and December. Aside from sales and planning for the year ahead, I always had quite a lot of time on my hands, something I was not used to. For the first two Januaries in business, I went back to online dating. Nothing really became of it each time, a few dates and not much else. My heart wasn't really in it anymore, I found my business so much more fulfilling and it was so personal to be working towards something I had created. There was nothing quite like it.

After the third Christmas and into my third year of trading, I was feeling exhausted. I had also got involved in a friendship that had been born out of business which was turning sour. Through mutual shared experiences, which I had moved on from but the other person had not, I found myself being triggered with my old stuff with my family. As I was really sensitive, I found I was soaking up the negative energies of the other person and feeling it as my own. I supported the friend but in the end I had to distance myself as it became unhealthy and stuff was projected onto me. Since my intense counselling years ago, I was much better at recognising when this was happening and had learnt how to hand stuff back that wasn't mine. I think that this coupled with the physical and mental exhaustion was overwhelming and I got very low for a while.

I went to see a mentor that another friend had recommended which really helped me to see how unbalanced my life had become. She was also shocked to discover that I had taken strong anti depressant medication for my entire adult life. With encouragement and very slow weaning I started to come off of the tablets. I had attempted a few times over the years and got so far before turning into a blubbering mess and unable to function with daily life. The physical side effects of weaning off were very severe with the worst feeling being a weird sensation in your head, as though your brain was tremoring. I saw my GP and they agreed also. I had come to terms with taking it as my doctor had once said to treat it as thought a diabetic takes their insulin and needs it. I accepted this but now this mentor had challenged me, and I felt in a much better place mentally to do it. My mum had always felt concerned at my taking them and I had done a lot of research. Many cases were recorded of people taking this drug and becoming addicted long term, and when they attempted to stop, however slow the process, they relapsed. There were also questions raised over the long term effects on a person's body and mind of taking the drug. I reduced incredibly slowly over the span of around a year, cutting the lowest tablets into quarters to eliminate any bad effects. I was fine for most of the year and was very proud of being on only a minute dose after all of this time. I wanted to feel how I would be as well without the powerful chemicals in my system. Then, I began to change, and feel different. I went downhill pretty fast and was crying for no reason every day. My thoughts were jumbled and I felt very anxious. I stood it for as long as I could as I was so determined to be drug free. It had been a tough journey also to quit and I did not want to let all of that hard work go to waste, but after a couple more weeks of feeling bad and worse, I relented. I refused to take a strong dose as before though and kept on a lower dose. My mood and thoughts soon started to balance out again. However at this moment in my life, I was not ready to make any vast changes regarding my business as I still felt I had more to achieve and I could not take my foot off of the pedal just yet. I did start to have little doubts over what I was seeking and doing though. I did go at a bit of a slower pace. I was also referred to the hospital as I was experiencing difficulty with my breathing and having episodes where my heart would beat very fast, even when resting. Each time I was told to slow down my lifestyle and I was given physio to do for dysfunctional breathing. The breathing pattern I had got into was impacting on my body in other ways too and I experienced significant neck pain which was very troublesome.

I was always reading, still keen to learn more about psychology and business and ways of self improvement. There were always webinars I wanted to see and podcasts to hear and books to read.

Joe was invited to London to take part in an achievers award event, one proud mum went along by his side. We both got the chance to meet Levi Roots, a foodie entrepreneur, afterwards and we got a photo to remember the special day by. Later that year, Joe made the transition from high school to college this year after getting excellent exam results. He was the top of his school in Maths, what a proud moment. Times to treasure.

I became very restless within my business and lost some of my passion which fuelled me. I had done a fair amount of speaking at networking events and at women's groups about my business journey which always was based on my "why". As each talk passed, I became increasingly aware that all I wanted to do was to tell my story. My business no longer felt enough for me, I knew I had much deeper work to share with the world.

CHAPTER TWENTY FOUR
RESTLESS

It's funny how things happen in life, how one happening leads to another to another. I often pondered over this and asked myself many big questions about life itself. People, life and why things happen fascinated me.

I had a lot to ask myself at this moment in time. How was I to share my story? Would I be accepted? Would anybody care? Whom would I be talking to? How would it help? The questions went on and on.

I was writing, journalling sporadically. I worked best with my instinct, my intuition and with my energy flow.

Before it was time for the annual Christmas sales season, I went to see a speaker that was recommended to me in London. I did some research and loved her energy. That day, a lot changed for me. I was never the same again. It was a very compelling and full on day, charged with energy and emotion. It was such a powerful experience that I made two big decisions that day. The first was that I was going to quit my business and the second was that I was going to become a speaker. I was convinced that I could learn from this amazing lady speaker, I resonated with so much that was shared that day. With this big shift, came much heart felt emotion and I sobbed. Tears of relief of admitting to myself that I did not want to carry on with my business but also grieving at that thought. It was like a baby, my first business and all of the love and nurture it had received. There was no going back, the decision was made and I was also excited to be moving forward.

I found myself rushing to the back of the room to be one of the first to sign up to the Speaker training, I didn't even know the exact details except that I had to do it. It was a lot of money for me at the time so I paid with a credit card that I used in business. I was congratulated afterwards by several people in the room, people that had already done the training. I was thrilled to find out that the training was going to be in Portugal at the start of the following year. I felt impatient at wishing it was sooner as I was enthused at my sudden decisions. The journey home on the train was exhausting, as the day's emotions caught up with me. I never did things by halves.

On waking the following day, I immediately felt a wondrous and elated feeling. It grew into the most intense feeling of gratitude I had ever experienced in my life. This lasted solidly for two weeks. I cannot describe fully the level at which it was felt, as I had never felt this before. The only way in which I could get close to how I felt was that if I were to be religious, that I had found God. I elatedly told my family and close friends of my decisions. I found myself doing the most random acts of kindness, I remember that I gave away free jewellery from my stock to a stranger at an event as I felt her pain. I kept experiencing amazingness in the forms of people and happenings that were brought to me. It was an incredible fortnight, then it subsided somewhat to a more usual level.

I slowly began to recognise that the business mission I had been on was not only about proving to myself that I could achieve the "successful life" I had always aspired to, but the real reason why. I was so ashamed of myself, of my past, of my struggle for years in and out of jobs like a yoyo, lengthy periods of being on sickness benefit and of being in a very dark place. The shame was accompanied by guilt. However, I was also becoming a lot more connected to my heart again and the deep desire I felt to help others.

Christmas came and went, by the time the seasonal sales were over I was so exhausted, the forth year running. Two thirds of the business's profit was made in six weeks of the year so it was exceptionally busy with little time for rest.

I spent most of January resting and preparing myself for my trip and training in Portugal at the end of the month. I was excited but also had little doubts and niggles. I was a very analytical person after years of therapy and self reflection that I had been through and could sometimes be prone to over thinking.

On arriving at the destination it was the most magnificent hotel and grounds. Very contemporary but very luxurious. The words "a millionaire's playground" sprang to mind. The room I was sharing was beautiful and the food was delicious. So much choice and beautifully presented, the chef in me approved enormously.

I felt excited for the following day when the course would start, and I hardly slept in anticipation.

Day one was great and I was pumped with energy, I did become emotional at one point when I recognised how proud I felt of myself for getting to this point. I had not come with a clear business idea which made the learning more challenging and I did find it muddled and struggled at times to follow, my brain didn't like it. That night I could barely sleep as my mind was so active.

The next day it all changed for me. I no longer felt any warmth from the speaker trainer and it was a cold hard sell. My initial feeling was anger. I was angry to be sold to when I had not even received what I had paid for. We are not talking pocket money either. It was sell, sell, sell and I felt like a sucker. I had anticipated there would be sales of course, it was a business event, but not like this.

The presentation was also very muddled and not in any order as it was in our workbooks and I found it very hard to follow. I became very emotional and very detached as I realised that this was not what I was about or wanted to do within my business or to other people. I felt strongly against it as it felt dishonest to me. I spoke to several members of the team but found it not very helpful and I sobbed openly. There were a few others upset also. This was really not what I had imagined. I really wanted to go home. I felt sickened to be a part of it. I had a calling to help people with mental health struggles and without them having to hand over a large sum of money. I genuinely cared. This felt so very manipulative. To be taught to tap into peoples emotions to gain money, to follow a tried and tested strategy, felt wrong on every level. When you have spent the most part of your life struggling with your own emotions, to be deliberately manipulating someone else's felt awful. I don't know how, but I stayed in the room for the duration of the day, in between crying bouts. My first impressions of this speaker had changed. How could I learn from someone that I did not trust nor agree with? I couldn't.

My feelings created some friction between myself and my room mate, as she felt differently to me. I was exhausted after getting upset, not sleeping and fighting against the day. I wanted to clear my mind. I decided I would not be finishing the last day, it was not for me at all. I felt really homesick and just longed to be home and feel okay again. I barely slept again that night, so in four days I had only had ten hours of sleep. My mind was alert through the much distress.

It brought about all kinds of other feelings, like disappointment too and concern over the money I had invested for this. God I was furious.

I stayed in my room the following morning and I was called on the phone. They tried to cajole me into attending but I was having none of it and told them clearly that it was not my cup of tea. I spoke to a couple of friends back in England which helped and one said that she too had felt very similar after attending this event. I didn't feel quite as alone then. I met my room mate for lunch and seized the opportunity to speak with the trainer's husband. He did not know what to say to me and offered me bonuses worth x amount. I looked at him in disbelief, they just put a money tag on everything. I said that I wanted a refund and he could see how upset I was. I was to leave it with him.

The departure time could not arrive quickly enough, I was desperate to get away from that place and get home. I was very fortunate to share the airport transport with a lovely lady which did happen by chance after her taxi had left early. We shared experiences of the stay and she also was not feeling great. It was a relief to talk to someone who understood.

I must have resembled a zombie at the airport and could hardly think straight with the sleep deprivation and stress. I felt very anxious all of the flight home and when I finally arrived home, my mum and Joe were shocked at how I was. It all tumbled out, my experience and I cried with relief to be home again. I slept like a log that night in my own bed again.

After resting the following day, I then sent an email to the speaker and her company. For weeks, I was both ignored and then offered other products and a chance to attend the next event. I was very clear in asking for a refund as per their guarantee. They were not wanting to honour this. In no uncertain terms did I want a repeat performance. After about two months of writing letters, emails and phone calls I got a solicitor's advice. She told me what I had suspected, that their legal papers had nothing in it of any value in these circumstances. Only when I told them that I was going to take legal action did they sit up and take notice. Within an hour or two I had several emails and the first from the actual speaker in the whole saga. I was disgusted at how they treated me and their customer service said it all. I got my refund. Result – at last some justice.

I could not wait to put the last two months behind me and move on as it had been very draining and taken me away from my normal self.

I was uncertain of my future and what I would do but I embarked on some voluntary mentoring with two organisations for disadvantaged young people. I loved this work and it was very rewarding. From this came a few people approach me to ask for business mentoring and support. I had a few clients but I wanted something that focussed more on mindset and peoples feelings.

I did some more speaking. I tried a couple of other projects and people to work with but nothing felt right. I realised that trying to work with others that did not share the same values was not going to work, there was too much conflict.

CHAPTER TWENTY FIVE
LETTING GO

Sitting in a café one day after meeting a business friend, I began to make notes for a new talk that I was writing. Before long, the notes had become fifty plus pages about my life journey in brief. I guess this was the start of this book.

I tried a couple more different ventures during this year, all ending in the same way, leaving a bad taste in my mouth. I had to work on my own project and I could set the level of integrity and work by my values important to me. You could never accuse me of sitting back and doing nothing that's for sure, I was always taking action and had a lot of drive.

Halfway through the year, I began what felt like a natural letting go process. Letting go of things, happenings and people that no longer served me.

I talked more and very openly on social media about my experiences with my mental and emotional health over time, and about ways in which I had helped myself. My natural "entertainer" showed itself when I made a series of videos about different topics that were important to me. Through this, I actually had some family choose to disown me, they could not accept what I was doing and did not understand my reasons. I also let some friends go that were not supportive of me any longer.

It was a very challenging year. I had a couple of buyers for my business but both pulled out. It was not meant to be.

I felt more and more focussed on the desire to help others, especially with my ongoing mentoring and seeing my clients progress. It was born from deep within my soul, right back to the place where I had felt so desperate in my darkest times and the empathy I felt for others in that place.

I started to build on my previous studies and embarked on a coaching course but I soon peeled back from that as it was not what I felt would help people whom had been through similar experiences such as I, it felt as though it were scratching the surface more than getting very deep to the crux of a problem.

I spent hours and hours and hours reading and researching, and it always came back to the same thought, I had to share my story as this is what had helped me so much over the years, reading about other's struggles that I could identify with. As I had never found one source of therapy that had helped me on its own. Medication suppressed a lot of feelings and treated the symptoms and not the cause. So hearing of what others did or did not do was huge. So I began to formulate my book idea more and planned a structure with actual chapters based on my own life's time-line. It felt a lot more real and when I first began to write a chapter it did feel amazing and a release.

Through social media I had a mental health/inspirational

publishing agent connect with me and after discussion, I was wildly spurred on to write more. I went to visit the company and the owner and was invited to send in more chapters as they liked my writing style.

I struggled with keeping the focus as I had fears about money and survival take over me, old triggers as I knew that next year things would change for me financially with no longer having a child of a certain age in A Level education.

I was living through bouts of fear and great passion and excitement on a regular basis and no I was not bipolar. The next few months were really hard and I hit some lows. When the fear was at its worst I felt paralysed with it and went into big panics. Then I would be calm again. It was an exhausting cycle. After investing quite a lot of money into various trainings I realised it was all already within me if I slowed down long enough to hear, see and feel it.

I wanted to face some of the remaining fears I had as a challenge to myself, that were not business related. In a short space of time, I held a snake, a giant stick insect (the tarantula's in the store were too venomous) and laid on a bed of nails with the photos to prove it. That felt amazing to do those things.

I recognised that a lot of my tears were also tears of grief at the thought of my son leaving for university next year. I went through cycles of being inconsolable to calm with that as the waves of loss washed over me. There was a lot going on.

Joe, his dad and I attended many different university open days and at the last one, I could not hold back some tears. Whilst I did not want to upset Joe or make him feel bad in any way I was struggling to contain my feelings. Loss came from loving so much and I really love Joe so much. I wouldn't have had it any other way as I wanted him to be happy, healthy and thriving as he was but it did not take away the sad loss I was already feeling. Other symptoms I had when I was experiencing anxiety was an irritated bladder and a very sore oesophagus region. I took medication for both which helped a little but sometimes they were extremely aggravated. I had lost control of my bladder on occasion when I was really wound up. I felt like a freak with all of the shameful things I felt and experienced. That may sound harsh but it was how I felt.

With lots more reading, I had more and more insights into my lifelong behaviours and emotions and thoughts. I took weeks off of not working in the run up to Christmas and listened quietly to myself, with no-one else advising me or telling me this strategy or that step to follow. I felt done with the business world as I knew it and needed to follow my way only with little other guidance.

Finances were tight with not working but I was determined to have a holiday with my son as in the summer we only managed a few days away. Joe was talking about possibly holidaying with his friends next summer so I thought we would treat ourselves before Christmas and escape the seasonal mayhem whilst we were at it. I booked us a week away to the canary island of Fuerventura and it was so lovely to spend quality time with Joe. We had many laughs and conversations, and most days we played scrabble sitting in a café bar. It was magical. I did a lot more thinking whilst away and writing my book was the top thought along with setting up a new venture in the new year, based on my learnings from my life.

Chapter Twenty Six

Reinventing Myself Again

Christmas and New Year of 2016 was quiet and relaxing, very relaxing in fact. I spent hours and hours watching films and box sets on Netflix, switching off from my worries and retraining myself to relax. It was bliss. I had used to enjoy a gripping film or drama pre-business but had not allowed myself any time much to partake in such relaxing activities in the last four years. In hindsight, I had been very tough on myself, but I did what I thought was right at the time. What more can you do?

Thoughts for the new year were to start afresh. Terminate my first business and sell off all of the stock, clear my business debt that had accumulated, get my book written and published and create an online business in self development, my big passion.

I started out with great intentions but soon came across

stumbling blocks. Something did not feel right on a deep level. I spent a month really struggling to dig deep and unearth what was bothering me, all of the time feeling worried sick about my having little income. It was a very difficult month to get through, I did endless reading and researching about all kinds of topics that I felt drawn to. Spiritual awakening, trauma, various mental disorders, business burnout to name a few. I felt that they all had a place in what I was currently going through and of who I was or part of me. The burnouts were the consequence of my personality – the deep feelings of passion I felt and the all or nothing thinking I had. I never knew when to stop once I was in the throes of passion for my work. It always became all consuming, finding balance in life was the ultimate struggle for me.

I advertised my business to sell and had some interest but nothing became of it, the universe was indicating that there was a reason. Maybe it was too personal to my own story and was not meant to belong to anyone else.

Something kicked in within me, and I set to work on my book. Within eleven days I had written the bulk part. The words just flooded out of me and flowed onto the page. I went on a journey through my life and recalled memories that I had not known were in my head. Over forty thousand words and I was nearing the end. It felt such a release and I could feel shame leaving me that had been held prisoner in my mind and heart for a long time. Some parts triggered more emotions than others but the end was in sight and I was determined to publish this book.

I felt as though I wanted to do some further training, always wanting to learn and help both myself and others more. I looked into counsellor training but soon came to realise that I had to remain anonymous to do that. I believed in the power of sharing your story so I came away from that idea. I did some training on anxiety and critical thinking which was excellent.

I began to feel as though my life was falling into place again after a very unsettled period. I had weathered the storm and actually come through it shining this time. I had also embarked on an exercise and healthy eating plan after gaining weight since I had started my business journey some four and a half years ago. It was in a healthy way, no faddy diets or strict regimes. That was also a sign that I had come such a long way. For years after recovering from my bulimia I still had a tight hold over my calorie consumption which kept my weight stable but also it was very harsh. Hopefully now I could relax a little more and focus on the nutritional aspects of food rather than the calorific value and my weight loss or gain.

Coming up towards the end of February 2017 as I write this chapter, I feel full of hope for the future.

CHAPTER TWENTY SEVEN

IT ALL MAKES SENSE

Writing this book itself has been very healing, a superb therapy process. It has been amazing to fulfil one of my life long ambitions of becoming an author. It has also been the chrysalis to confirm my solid realisations, truths, insights and learnings.

I have written this book as myself, as I was at each stage, capturing how I thought and felt at the time. As I go through my life's journey I am going to reflect and share with you my insights as the forty six year old woman I am today.

If this were to inspire or help another person to shed some insight on their own self then that would be incredible and I also see this book as my big hug to anyone suffering right now. I know all too well what it feels like to feel alone in the world, struggling with painful thoughts and emotions and I want you to know that I care and that you are not alone.

Let's begin.

Having to leave my friends, changing homes and schools a few times actually taught me about leaving my comfort zone and resilience. We never grow as a person if we try to control everything in our lives to stay the same.

My parents – my dad greatly inspired me with his work ethic and to believe in himself enough to have the courage to work for himself, to follow his passion and earn a good living from doing what he loved. My mum, so sweet, kind and caring, always wanting to help others. They both taught me that self care is vital and must come before any other love for another. They did not always do this for themselves, nor I for a long time.

Some of my struggles were normal teenage issues. I may have missed some of them out at that age and experienced them at a later stage, but it helped me enormously to raise my own son. The bullying, at all ages, has made me aware that the real issue is not about me, but about the bully. To remember not to take attacks like these personally and aim to give forgiveness to the other person as they must be struggling themselves and have a need to control and put down another being to make themselves feel better.

Being told I was quiet, boring, fat, ugly etc – made me change, but then to recognise as I have explained above, but also that we all have a core personality and just because it is different to others does not make it wrong in any way. I have gone back to being the true me.

Feeling a "misfit" or a loner or not fitting in, this was about me being me, understanding and not being afraid to be individual.

Sadly, that schools and health professionals are still not dealing effectively with issues such as bullying, mental health, trauma.

As I matured, I became more and more self aware. I understood myself a lot better and that a part of my personality was very sensitive. On research, I recognised myself as a Highly Sensitive Person or an Empath, but labelling is not always a helpful thing to do. Being highly sensitive, made me feel everything on a deep level, be it good or bad. To control these emotions was very challenging. I also had much empathy for others that were in pain, enough to motivate me to do something in my lifetime to help. To also be aware, of feeling others "stuff", their emotions and knowing how to separate the two, which to this day is a work in progress.

People, and my parents in particular, were doing the best they could, at that time, with what they had. Understanding this was paramount in my forgiveness and letting go of anger and hurt towards them for what I had not received when I needed it as a young girl. They loved me dearly but were hurting themselves. Unhealthy habits, if not nipped in the bud, can continue for generation after generation.

A person's appearance, or weight, is not based on their worth. It is just a small part of their being and what the world can first see. By being introverted and secretive in nature, taught me to speak up and become more assertive. To not allow others to use me and to go after what I wanted for myself without feeling guilty or greedy.

The importance of family and of close friends and ultimately of love and connection. If we are not feeling these vital energies then we seek love and connection elsewhere and sometimes in unhealthy choices such as through addictions. It does have to start first and foremost with the love you have for yourself. We all seek to belong, to feel familiarity, normal behaviour. To form healthy connections with others.

Life can change in an instant, we need to stay true to ourselves and it will all be okay when we have a solid sense of whom we are rather than changing ourselves to fit in with others.

To tune into your own true passions, such as writing creatively, psychology and understanding people and the mind. Our passions are what makes us and if we can harness these to create a life we love. Exams and further study are not the only paths in life, especially true for more creative minds.

Learn how to be quiet within, through meditation or just being still, to listen to your inner self and to trust it, as that self knows the answers for you.

To not attempt to read other's minds. I don't actually know what they are thinking, and by assuming or guessing can create a whole set of new problems. Ask, find out the truth and go from there.

Everyone has some form of stress in their lives, and finding a healthy way to release any negative feelings, so they are not able to build up.

If the going gets tough, ask for help, however hard it may be. Be brave as it is not a sign of weakness as I once believed.

Whether it be an illness or a problem in life, aim to investigate and treat the cause rather than the symptom to stop it in its tracks.

That being unheard is one of the most hardest feelings to cope with. I try to listen to others and give that respect.

I found that loss and bereavement is not only exclusive to losing people in your life. Grieving for what you missed out on, but at the same time, asking yourself how you can grieve something that you never had?

In order for change to take place, we have to create it by making smaller changes. It may sound obvious but can be easy to get stuck in a cycle of wanting a different outcome but to keep doing the same actions.

I used my vivid imagination, which may have been both a blessing and a curse, to create myself coping strategies. What could you create for yourself to help you with?

A thought is just a thought, and that it is us that attaches a feeling to it. Just realising this helped me to analyse my thoughts much more to detach some of the emotion and recognise that it was not real.

By avoiding and procrastinating issues or problems or simply things to do, we can further problems. Tackle each separate point one at a time to avoid overwhelm.

The futility of comparison. So easy to do and it serves no purpose other than to punish ourselves. Realise that everyone is individual and on their own path with different experiences. How can you possibly compare when you understand that?

Set yourself aims and goals, for either obtaining something that you want in life or to overcome something. Create a step by step plan and take the action.

You can do so much to help yourself. A good starting point is to become aware of your thoughts, feelings and behaviours. Then ask yourself why you think what you think and why you do what you do.

Sometimes we need to reach rock bottom, or a low, to realise that we do not want that for ourselves anymore in order to create change.

That what we have in our lives is ultimately what we have attracted to us by our own thoughts and what we focus on mostly. This can be anything and be negative and positive.

That we are all responsible for our own happiness. We cannot look or expect others or outside influences make us happy. We have to look deep within and find it for ourselves. Then do that.

To not allow feelings of fear to stop us moving forward. A lot of fear is based on old beliefs and old feelings of fear. Sit quietly, question it and see what comes up.

Life is about balance, I truly believe we are here to enjoy ourselves and feel love and joy. Balance out the serious times with fun.

I also spent much time studying the mind and what happens

when it has experienced deep trauma, especially as a young person in the developmental years. It made such sense to me and was actually a big relief to recognise a lot of my "symptoms" through the impact trauma has on the brain, on the cortex and limbic systems. I'm no doctor, but knowing how this can create, impulsiveness (I am incredibly so!), responding excessively to minor triggers (this has been known to happen many times...), a poor working memory which makes tasks that involve lots of instructions for example much harder (the main reason I never learnt to drive) . Also your whole being can remain in a fight or flight state, which triggers the body to produce excessive cortisol. The cortisol can wreak havoc on the body and mind creating illness and prolonging the problems.

Overall, I came to the conclusion that everything was a combination of my personality, my genes, my experiences in life. I am truly grateful for what it has taught me, despite of the pain. Most of all, to have hope for better things. Through hope comes positivity, and I became very determined and out of my stubbornness came tenacity to never give up trying.

The Invisible Girl